康复专业
英语基础读本

［美］刘浩　主编

ESSENTIAL ENGLISH FOR
REHABILITATION AND THERAPY
PROFESSIONALS

U0397797

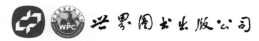
世界图书出版公司

上海·西安·北京·广州

图书在版编目（CIP）数据

康复专业英语基础读本 /（美）刘浩主编 . —上海：
上海世界图书出版公司，2020.1（2020.11重印）
　ISBN 978-7-5192-6819-0

　Ⅰ. ①康… Ⅱ. ①刘… Ⅲ. ①康复—英语 Ⅳ.
①R493

中国版本图书馆CIP数据核字（2019）第223087号

书　　名	康复专业英语基础读本	
	Kangfu Zhuanye Yingyu Jichu Duben	
主　　编	[美] 刘　浩	
责任编辑	胡冬冬	
装帧设计	南京展望文化发展有限公司	
出版发行	上海世界图书出版公司	
地　　址	上海市广中路88号9–10楼	
邮　　编	200083	
网　　址	http://www.wpcsh.com	
经　　销	新华书店	
印　　刷	上海颛辉印刷厂有限公司	
开　　本	787 mm× 1092 mm　1/16	
印　　张	7	
字　　数	100 千字	
版　　次	2020 年 1 月第 1 版　　2020 年 11 月第 2 次印刷	
书　　号	ISBN 978–7–5192–6819–0/R·524	
定　　价	60.00 元	

编写人员

主 编　刘　浩

参编者（按姓氏笔画排序）

方蓓苓　乔鸿飞　全莉娟　刘　浩　李　盈　李应志

张　松　张　鹏　陆玉瑾　赵明明　郭媛媛　温子星

PREFACE

前　言

In the last 10 years, rehabilitation medicine in China has developed quicker than many people ever imagined. Rehabilitation therapy colleges or departments have sprung up all over China. As a new medical specialty, many foreign rehab experts have been invited from abroad to China to give presentations, symposia, workshops, and training classes in English. The topics cover almost all aspects of subspecialties of rehabilitation medicine and therapy. During this time, a lot of rehab equipment, instruments, and devices have been imported from outside China; they contain user guides, manuals or instructions written in English. In addition, more and more rehab professionals and students travel to other countries to study rehabilitation medicine and therapy as visiting scholars or international students, they have to communicate in English with their professors, mentors or fellow classmates. With all of these said, it is imperative for rehabilitation professionals from China to have sufficient English proficiency to communicate efficiently with foreign rehab counterparts.

Currently students in rehab therapy programs in China are studying English in Medicine

在过去的10年中，中国的康复医学发展得比许多人想象的要快得多。康复治疗学院或系如雨后春笋般涌现。作为一门新的医学专业，这些年许多外国康复专家被邀请到中国用英语进行专业演讲、研讨会、工作坊和培训班。他们的讲课主题几乎涵盖了康复医学和治疗专业的所有方面。在此期间，国内从国外也进口了许多康复设备、仪器和器具，以及所含带的用英语编写的用户指南、手册或说明。此外，越来越多的康复专业人士和学生作为访问学者或留学生前往其他国家学习康复医学和治疗，他们不得不用英语与他们的教授、导师或同学进行交流。所有这些都表明，中国的康复从业人员必须具备足够的专业英语水平，才能与外国康复同行进行有效的沟通。

目前，国内康复治疗院系的学生学习的专业英语是医学院

instead of English in rehabilitation therapy. This may cause therapy students to have challenges in listening, speaking, reading, and writing rehab-related English.Thus, a book with more rehab terms and jargon is needed, which may provide some help for these students.

The author of this book is a physical therapy professor who earned his PhD in Human Anatomy and practiced as a licensed therapist for many years in the United States. As we know. Anatomy, kinesiology, and physiology are the three most fundamental courses for rehab therapy students and professionals, so the main content of this book is in anatomy, but with some emphasis on kinesiology and physiology. To make it convenient for Chinese readers, each of the book's 16 chapters or lessons include: text in English, new words with Chinese translation, 5 multiple choice questions related to the text, Chinese translation of the text, and audio-recording of the text in English. It should be noted that the audio-recording is recorded by a native English speaker.

Based on the contents, this book can be used by rehab therapy students and professionals, anatomy instructors and international students in medicine, sports medicine specialists, and even medical professionals.

学生用的医学英语，而不是康复治疗英语。这就可能会导致治疗系的学生在听、说、读、写康复相关的英语方面遇到挑战。因此，需要一本具有更多康复术语和行话的书，以便为这些学生提供一些帮助。

本书的主编是在美国获得人体解剖学博士学位的物理治疗系教授。众所周知，解剖学、运动学和生理学是康复治疗系学生和专业人士的3个最基础的课程，因此本书的主要内容是解剖学，但会有一些侧重于运动学和生理学的内容。为了方便中国读者，本书的16个课程包括：英文课文、生词中文翻译、与课文内容相关的5个选择题、课文的中文翻译以及课文的英语录音。应该提一下的是，课文的英语录音是由母语为英语的人朗读录制的。

根据内容，本书可供康复治疗学生和专业人士，解剖学教师和学医的留学生，运动医学专家，甚至医学专业人士使用。

CONTENTS

目 录

Medical Terminology—How a Medical Word is Made Up

医学术语——医学词汇是怎样构成的

1

Students who study rehabilitation medicine and therapy in English often find out that medical terms are one of the major obstacles for them to move forward. Even students whose native language is English will often feel that studying medical terminology is like studying another language. This is because most medical terms are jargons that are not used by the general public and are not commonly spoken during our daily life.

Actually, medical terminology may not be as hard to study as you think. When deciphering medical terms, you may find that a lot of them are rooted from either Latin or Greek language. Latin roots are usually used to describe anatomical structures. For example, in anatomy a nerve that innervates skin is often called a "cutaneous nerve". For example, the medial cutaneous nerve of the arm is the nerve that innervates the medial side of the arm. Here, the root word "cutane" indicates skin in Latin. On the other hand, Greek roots are used to describe a disease, treatment, diagnosis, or

使用英语进行康复医学及康复治疗技术的学习时，学习者会发现医学术语是他们前进路上的主要障碍之一。即使是那些以英语为母语的学生也经常感觉学习医学术语几乎是在学习另外一门语言，因为大多数医学专有词往往不被公众应用，也不会在我们的日常生活中经常使用。

实际上医学术语可能没有你想象的那么难。如果你深入解读一些医学词汇，你就会发现许多术语是以拉丁语或希腊语为词根。拉丁词根经常用来描述解剖结构，例如，在解剖学中，支配皮肤的神经，我们经常称它为"cutaneous nerve"，如"medial cutaneous nerve of arm"是指支配手臂内侧的神经。这里的"cutane"就是拉丁语中皮肤的意思。另一方面，希腊词根被用来描述某种疾病、疗法、诊

condition. For example, when we refer to the condition where a nerve innervates a specific skin area in relation to a spinal segment, it is often called a "dermatome". For example, the dermatome for the 10th thoracic spinal segment is a belt-like nerve distribution around the umbilicus (also known as the belly button). Here, the root word "dermato" indicates skin in Greek.

An element placed before or after the stem is called a prefix or a suffix. A prefix describes a number, time, position/location, direction, or negation, while a suffix indicates a pathological (disease or abnormality) symptom, surgical procedure, or part of speech. For example, biceps (a muscle with two heads: bi—two, ceps—heads); arthritis (joint inflammation: arthr—joint, itis—inflammation), myalgia (muscle pain: my—muscle, algia—pain); subcutaneous (below the skin: sub—below, cutaneous—skin); contralateral (opposite side: contra—opposite, lateral—side), ipsilateral (same side: ipsi—same, lateral—side), mastectomy (mast—breast, ectomy—removal).

As you can see from these examples, many medical terms are "constructed" from a combination of two-word parts (prefix + suffix) or three-word parts (prefix + stem + suffix). When another root word or a suffix that starts with a consonant is added to the stem, a vowel must be used to connect the word parts. This is called a "combining vowel", and is usually an "o, i, or e". For example, kinesiology (science in motion:

断或状态。例如，当我们指某个与脊髓节段相关的皮肤区域的神经支配时，我们往往称它为"dermatome"。举个例子，第10对胸神经节段（the dermatome for the 10th thoracic spinal segment）指的是第10对胸神经相对应的皮神经支配，这里的dermato就是指希腊语中的皮肤。

像上述的词根一样可以被放在词干或后的要素叫作前缀或后缀。前缀描述数字、时间、位置、方向或表否定，而后缀则指病理（疾病或异常）症状、外科手术过程或是发炎的一部分。例如，biceps（有两个肌腹或肌头的肌肉：bi—两个，ceps—头部）；arthritis（关节炎：arthr—关节，itis—炎症）；myalgia（肌肉疼痛：my—肌肉的，algia—疼痛）；subcutaneous（皮下的：sub—下面的，cutaneous—皮肤的）；contralateral（对侧：contra—相对的，对面的，lateral——侧）；ipsilateral（同侧：ipsi—相同的，lateral——侧）；mastectomy（乳房切除术：mast—乳房，ectomy—切除术）。

从上面的例子中可以看出，许多医学词汇都是由两个单词部分（前缀+后缀）或是三个部分（前缀+词干+后缀）组合而成的。当一个带有辅音开头的词干或后缀要与一个前缀连接时，必须用一个元音字母来连接这两个部分，这就是"连接元音"，经常使用字母o、i或e。举个例子：kinesiology（运动学：kinesi—

kinesi–motion; logy–science, combining vowel–o). sternocleidomastoid (stern–chest, cleid–clavicle, mastoid–small process behind the ear, combining vowel–o). myositis (muscle inflammation, my–muscle, sitis–inflammation, combining vowel–o).

To determine the meaning of a medical term, you may need to understand the meaning of the prefix, stem (if available), and suffix before you can understand the meaning of the whole word. Rehabilitation professionals face patients mainly with dysfunctions in neurological, musculoskeletal, cardiovascular, and other systems. A few tables of root words, their definitions, and examples with a focus on those that rehabilitation professionals may see during their everyday practice are presented below.

运动, logy—科学, 连接元音—o); sternocleidomastoid(胸锁乳突肌: stern—胸部的, cleid—锁骨的, mastoid—乳头状突起, 连接元音—o); myositis(肌肉炎, my—肌肉的, sitis—炎症, 连接元音—o)。

为了确定一个医学词汇的含义, 在你搞懂整个词的含义之前, 你可能需要理解前缀、词干(如有的话)和后缀的含义。因为康复专业面对的主要是有神经、骨骼和肌肉或心血管等系统功能失调的患者, 因此我们提供几个表格, 表格中含有一些康复从业者在每天的实际工作中会见到的词根及其含义和举例。

Basic anatomy terms(基础解剖学术语)

Word(单词)	Meaning(解释)	Examples(举例)
abdominal 腹部的	abdomen 腹部	abdominal cavity 腹腔
lumbar 腰的	loin 腰部	quadratus lumborum 腰方肌
mammary 乳腺的	breast 乳房	mammary body 乳头体
nasal 鼻的	nose 鼻	nasal cavity 鼻腔
sternal 胸骨的	breastbone 胸骨	costosternal joint 胸骨关节
thoracic 胸的	chest 胸	thoracic cavity 胸腔
dorsal 背侧的	back 背侧的	dorsolateral 背外侧的
ventral 腹侧的	belly, anterior side of body 腹侧的	ventromedial 腹内侧的

Conditions（描述情形的前/后缀）

Prefix（前缀）	Meaning（解释）	Examples（举例）
ambi-	both 双侧的，两个的	ambidextrous 双手灵巧的
dys-	bad, painful, difficult 坏的，有障碍的，困难的	dyslexia 诵读困难；阅读障碍
eu-	good, normal 真的，好的，正常的	eukaryote 真核细胞
homo-	same 同样的	homogenous 同质的，同类的
iso-	equal, same 同一个的，相同的	isotope 放射性核素
mal-	bad, poor 坏的，不好的	malfunction 功能障碍
Suffix（后缀）	**Meaning（解释）**	**Examples（举例）**
-algia	pain 痛	myalgia 肌痛
-emia	blood 血	leukemia 白血病
-itis, sitis-	inflammation 炎症	nasitis, myositis 鼻窦炎，肌炎
-opathy	disease of ……的病	neuropathy 神经病
-pnea	breathing 呼吸的	dyspnea 呼吸困难

New words

terminology [ˌtɜːmɪˈnɒlədʒɪ] *n.* 术语

jargon [ˈdʒɑːɡən] *n.* 行话，术语

decipher [dɪˈsaɪfə(r)] *v.* 解读

cutaneous [kjʊˈteɪnɪəs] *adj.* 皮肤的

dermatome [ˈdɜːmətəʊm] *n.* 皮节感觉对应

innervate [ɪˈnɜːveɪt] *v.* 支配

spinal segment 脊柱节段

thoracic [θɔːˈræsɪk] *adj.* 胸的

belly [ˈbeli] *n.* 腹部

umbilicus [ʌmˈbɪlɪkəs] *n.* 肚脐

ipsilateral [ɪpsɪˈlætərəl] *adj.* 同侧的

prefix [ˈpriːfɪks] *n.* 前缀

suffix [ˈsʌfɪks] *n.* 后缀

negation [nɪˈɡeɪʃən] *n.* 否定

pathological [ˌpæθəˈlɒdʒɪkl] *adj.* 病理学的

abnormality [ˌæbnɔːˈmælətɪ] *n.* 异常

biceps [ˈbaɪseps] *n.* 二头肌

arthritis [ɑrˈθraɪtɪs] *n.* 关节炎

inflammation [ˌɪnfləˈmeɪʃən] *n.* 炎症

myalgia [maɪˈældʒə] *n.* 肌痛

subcutaneous [ˌsʌbkjʊˈtenjəs] *adj.* 皮下的

contralateral [kɒntrəˈlætərəl] *adj.* 对侧的

ipsilateral [ɪpsɪˈlætərəl] *adj.* 同侧的

mastectomy [mæˈstektəmɪ] *n.* 乳房切除术

consonant [ˈkɒnsənənt] *n.* 辅音

vowel [ˈvaʊəl] *n.* 元音

kinesiology [kɪˌniːsɪˈɒlədʒɪ] *n.* 运动学

sternocleidomastoid [ˈstərnɒˈklɪdmasˈtɔɪd] *n.* 胸锁乳突肌

mastoid [ˈmæstɔɪd] *n.* 乳突

myositis [maɪəʊˈsaɪtɪs] *n.* 肌炎

musculoskeletal [ˌmʌskjʊləʊˈskelətəl] *n.* 肌肉骨骼

cardiovascular [ˌkɑːdɪəʊˈvæskjələ(r)] *adj.* 心血管的

neuropathy [nʊˈrɒpəθɪ] *n.* 神经病

dyspnea [dɪsˈpniːə] *n.* 呼吸困难

------------------------------ **Questions** ------------------------------

1 Which one of the following word roots can be matched with " Cutane" in term of the same meaning?

A. Derm–　　　　　　　　　　B. Rostro–

C. Iso–　　　　　　　　　　　D. Quadra–

2 A muscle, which has four heads, is able to flex hip joint and powerfully extend the knee joint. This muscle is _____.

A. the quadratus femoris　　　　B. the quadriceps femoris

C. the quadratus lumborum　　　D. the biceps femoris

❸ After being initially evaluated, you notice that your physician writes down a term: Myalgia. What medical problem is he indicating?

A. Skin rash.　　　　　　　　　　　B. Muscle edema.

C. Muscle pain.　　　　　　　　　　D. Nerve numbness.

❹ Dr. Liu is a scientist that studies movement of human body. Which one of the following can appropriately describe who he is?

A. Kinesiologist.　　　　　　　　　　B. Biologist.

C. Anatomist.　　　　　　　　　　　D. Physiologist.

❺ Mr. Wang has been diagnosed of osteoarthritis. Based on what you learned, what is his medical problem?

A. Inflammation of bone marrow.　　B. Reduction of bone mass.

C. Inflammation of bone joint.　　　D. Tumor of bone surface.

Answers

❶ A　　❷ B　　❸ C　　❹ A　　❺ C

The Human Skeletal System
人体骨骼系统

2

The skeletal system is the framework of the human body and is formed by 206 bones in different sizes and shapes. These bones(Figure 2–1 and Figure 2–2) are connected to each other by joints. Each joint is stabilized by a joint capsule and surrounding accessory structures like ligaments, muscles, and retinacula. Most joints in the human body are synovial joints. In a synovial joint, the joint surface of two neighbouring bonesaresurroundedby the joint capsule. The inner structure of the capsule is comprised of the synovial membrane that provides synovial fluid to the joint for lubrication and nutrients. Outside the joint capsule, ligaments (except cruciate ligaments inside the knee joint) are tight connective tissue structures that cross a joint to ensure it is stable during movement activities. Muscles are soft tissue structures that cross one, two, or more joints and act to move the joint(s) in different directions. Retinacula are tight connective tissues as well, located in a joint area to stabilize the long

构建人体构架的骨骼系统由206块形状大小不一的骨头构成。这些骨骼（图2–1，图2–2）通过关节相互连接，每个关节通过关节囊和关节周围附属结构如关节周围韧带、肌肉和支持带固定。人体内大多数关节是滑膜关节，在一个滑膜关节内，两块相邻骨的关节面有关节囊包裹。关节囊的内层是可以为关节产生润滑液来提供润滑和营养物的滑膜。在关节囊的外面，韧带（膝关节交叉韧带这种囊内韧带除外）是跨过关节的致密结缔组织，以确保活动过程中关节的稳定性。肌肉作为一种软组织结构，跨过1个或2个关节，使关节在不同方向运动。肌肉支持带也是关节周围的致密结缔组织，在关节运动时稳固（跨过关节的）长条肌肉以免它们弓弦样膨出。

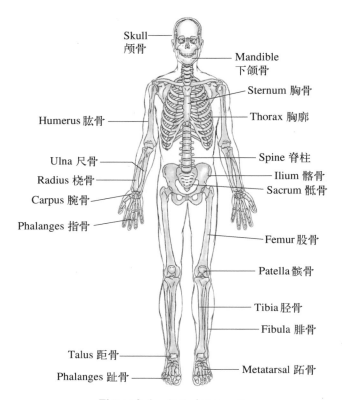

Skull
颅骨

Mandible
下颌骨

Sternum 胸骨

Humerus 肱骨

Thorax 胸廓

Ulna 尺骨

Spine 脊柱

Radius 桡骨

Ilium 髂骨

Carpus 腕骨

Sacrum 骶骨

Phalanges 指骨

Femur 股骨

Patella 髌骨

Tibia 胫骨

Fibula 腓骨

Talus 距骨

Phalanges 趾骨

Metatarsal 跖骨

Figure 2–1　Anterior aspect
（图2–1　前面观）

muscles and prevent them from bowstringing out during the joint movement.

　　The central part of the human skeleton is the vertebral column (also known as the spine) which is formed by five sections or levels of vertebral bones: cervical, thoracic, lumbar, sacral, and coccygeal. Together these five sections stack to make the curved vertebral column. The column connects with the skull rostrally, with the shoulder girdles and then the upper extremities anterosuperiorly, and with the pelvic girdle and then the lower extremities anteroinferiorly. Details of the

　　人体骨骼中心部分是脊椎（又称为脊柱），它包括五部分或节段的椎骨：颈椎、胸椎、腰椎、骶部和尾椎，这五部分椎骨堆叠在一起形成了弯曲的脊柱。脊柱与头颅骨相连，前上方与肩带及上肢相连，前下方与骨盆带及下肢相连。关于脊柱的细节将在下一节进行详细的描述。

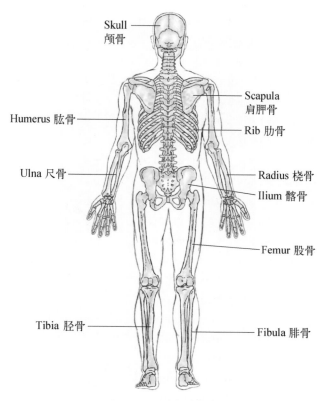

Figure 2–2   Posterior aspect
（图2-2   后面观）

vertebral column will be described in the next lesson.

The bones for the head and neck include primarily the skull, mandible, and hyoid bones. The skull is formed tightly by 22 cranial and facial bones. The skull articulates with the mandible through the temporomandibular joints bilaterally which act to move the jaw. The skull connects to the vertebral column through an articulation with the 1st cervical vertebrae. The hyoid bone is a small U-shaped bone floating between the chin and the thyroid cartilage and provides attachment spots for the

头颈部的骨骼主要包括头骨、下颌骨和舌骨。头骨由22块颅骨和面骨紧密连接而成，头骨通过颞下颌关节从两边与下颌骨相连来完成下颌运动，头骨同样通过与C1的关节和脊柱相连。舌骨是1块浮动在下巴和甲状软骨之间的U形骨骼，为支持吞咽和发音活动的舌骨上下肌群提供附着点。

suprahyoid and infrahyoid muscles to assist with swallowing and voice production.

The bones of the upper extremity connect with the trunk through the shoulder girdle which includes the scapula, sternum, clavicle, and proximal humerus. These 4 bones are linked through one non-synovial joint (the scapulothoracic), and three other synovial joints (the sternoclavicular joints, acromioclavicular joints, and glenohumeral joints). The glenohumeral joint articulates between the glenoid cavity of the scapula and the humeral head and is the main one of these four joints. When you raise your arm, the motion of the shoulder is the result of these four joints acting together. The distal humerus connects with the forearm through the elbow joint. The forearm includes two bones: the radius and the ulna, which further connects to the carpal bones through the wrist joint. In the hand, the metacarpal bones articulate with the carpal bones proximally and with the phalangeal bones distally. There are only two phalangeal bones for the thumb, while each of the other four fingers have three phalangeal bones: the proximal, middle, and distal phalanxes.

The bones of the lower extremity connect with the trunk through the pelvic girdle which includes the pelvic bone (sacrum + hip bone) and the femur. The hip joint is the main joint of the lower extremity that acts on the hipbone: the femoral head articulates with the acetabular fossa of the hipbone. At the distal part of the femur are the medial and lateral

　　上肢骨骼通过肩带与躯干相联系，肩带包括肩胛骨、胸骨、锁骨和肱骨近端。这4块骨骼通过一个非滑膜关节（肩胛胸壁关节）和其他3个滑膜关节（胸锁关节、肩锁关节和盂肱关节）相连接。盂肱关节由肩胛骨的关节盂和肱骨的肱骨头构成，是这4个关节中的主要关节。任何时候，当你举起你的手臂，肩关节的运动都需要这4个关节共同参与。肱骨远端通过肘关节与前臂相连，前臂包括2块骨：桡骨和尺骨，它们的远端通过腕关节与腕骨相连接。在手部，掌骨近端与腕骨相连，远端与指骨相连。拇指只有2节指骨，而其余4指每个手指都有3节指骨：近节指骨、中节指骨和远节指骨。

　　下肢骨通过骨盆带与躯干相连接，包括盆骨（骶骨＋髋骨）和股骨。髋关节是下肢与髋骨相连接的关节：股骨头与髋骨的髋臼相连接。股骨远端的内外侧髁与胫骨平台的内外侧髁相连接，需要指出的是位于股骨髁间窝的小骨头髌骨与股骨构成

epicondyles which articulate with the plateaus on both medial and lateral tibial condyles. It should be noted that a small bone called the patella is located in the intercondylar fossa of the femur to make the patellofemoral joint which aims to reduce the mechanical stress on the knee joint. Further down, the distal ends of both the tibia and fibula articulate with the proximal talus bone to make the ankle (talocrural) joint, in which the talus can fit snugly into the mortise-like space made by both the tibia and fibula. The distal talus articulates with the calcaneus bone through the subtalar joint. In the foot, the tarsal bones (including the navicular, cuneiform, and cuboid bones) articulate with the calcaneus proximally and with the metatarsal bones distally. The metatarsal bones then connect to the toes through metatarsophalangeal joints. During ambulation, the body weight can transfer all the way down through these lower extremity bones and joints to the feet, and vice versa. The reaction forces from the bottoms of both feet can travel back up to the trunk, even to the head and neck, traveling through all of the structures in between.

的髌股关节，可以起到减小膝关节机械应力的作用。再往下，胫骨和腓骨远端与距骨近端相连接形成踝关节（距小腿骨关节），其中距骨可以紧密填充由胫骨和腓骨所形成的榫状空间。距骨远端通过距下关节与跟骨相联系。足部区域，跗骨（包括舟骨、楔状骨和骰骨）的近端与跟骨相连接而远端则与跖骨相连接，跖骨可以通过跖趾关节与脚趾相联系。步行过程中，体重可以通过下肢骨骼及关节向下转移至足部；反之亦然，双脚底部的反作用力也可以通过这些骨性力学结构向上至躯干甚至头颈部。

New words

accessory [ək'sesərɪ] *adj.* 附属的，附加的
ligament ['lɪgəmənt] *n.* 韧带
retinacula [ˌretɪ'nækjʊlə] *n.* 支持带（retinaculum 的名词复数）
synovial joint　滑膜关节
synovial fluid　滑液

lubrication [ˌluːbrɪˈkeɪʃn] *n.* 润滑

nutrient [ˈnjuːtrɪənt] *n.* 营养物，营养品

cruciate ligaments　交叉韧带

vertebral column [ˈvəːtibrəlˈkɔləm] *n.* 脊柱

cervical [ˈsɜːvɪkl] *adj.* 颈的

thoracic [θɔːˈræsɪk] *adj.* 胸的

lumbar [ˈlʌmbə(r)] *adj.* 腰部的

sacral [ˈseɪkrəl] *adj.* 骶骨的

coccygeal [kɒkˈsɪdʒɪəl] *adj.* 尾骨的

curved [kɜːvd] *adj.* 弧形的，曲线的

skull [skʌl] *n.* 颅骨，头盖骨

rostral [ˈrɒstrəl] *adj.* 头端的，头侧的

shoulder girdle [ˈʃəʊldəˈgɜːdl] 肩带；肩带部

anterosuperiorly [æntəˈrəʊsuːprɪəlɪ] *adv.* 在前上方

pelvic girdle [ˈpelvɪkˈgɜːdl] 骨盆带

lower extremities 下肢

mandible [ˈmændɪbl] *n.* 下颚，下颚骨

articulate [ɑːˈtɪkjuleɪt] *v.* 与……关节连接

temporomandibular joints　颞下颌关节

bilaterally [ˌbaɪˈlætərəlɪ] *adv.* 两侧，双向地

thyroid cartilage [ˈθaɪrɔɪdˈkɑːtlɪdʒ] *n.* 甲状软骨

suprahyoid and infrahyoid muscles　舌骨上肌和舌骨下肌

scapula [ˈskæpjʊlə] *n.* 肩胛骨

sternum [ˈstɜːnəm] *n.* 胸骨

clavicle [ˈklævɪkl] *n.* 锁骨

proximal humerus [ˈprɔksiməlˈhjuːmərəs] 肱骨近端

sternoclavicular joints　胸锁关节

acromioclavicular joints　肩锁关节

glenohumeral joints　盂肱关节

radius and ulna　桡骨和尺骨

carpal bones　腕骨

metacarpal bones　掌骨

proximally [ˈprɒksɪməl] *adv.* 近端的

phalangeal bones 指骨

distally ['dɪstælaɪ] *adv.* 远侧的

sacrum ['seɪkrəm] *n.* 骶骨

femur ['fiːmə(r)] *n.* 股骨

acetabular fossa 髋臼窝

epicondyle [ˌepɪ'kɒndaɪl] *n.* 上髁

tibial condyle 胫骨髁

patella [pə'telə] *n.* 髌骨

intercondylar fossa 髁间窝

patellofemoral joint 髌股关节

tibia ['tɪbiə] *n.* 胫骨

talocrural joint 跗距关节

talus bone 距骨

calcaneus bone 跟骨

subtalar joint 距下关节

tarsal bones 跗骨

navicular [nə'vɪkjʊlə] bone 舟骨

cuneiform ['kjuːnɪfɔːm] *n.* 楔骨

cuboid bones 骰骨

metatarsal bones 跖骨

metatarsophalangeal joints 跖趾关节

vice versa [ˌvaɪs'vɜːsə] *adv.* 反之亦然

Questions

❶ The synovial fluid is able to provide lubrication and nutrients to the joint. Which of the following structures is responsible for producing the fluid?

A. The ligaments around the joint.

B. The retinacula around the joint.

C. The joint cartilage.

D. The synovial membrane of the joint capsule.

❷ There are five sections of vertebral bones. These sections are usually called:

A. cervical, thoracic, lumbar, sacral, and coccygeal.

B. cervical, thoracic, abdominal, sacral, and coccygeal.

C. cervical, thoracic, lumbar, pelvic, and coccygeal.

D. cervical, thoracic, abdominal, pelvic, and coccygeal.

❸ Which one of the bones below is always floating in the tissue and not articulated directly with any other bones?

A. The mandible.   B. The hyoid.

C. The first cervical vertebra.   D. The clavicle.

❹ There are four joints that are related to shoulder movement, like raising arms. Which one of these four joints is not a true synovial joint?

A. The scapulothoracic joint.   B. The sternoclavicular joint.

C. The acromioclavicular joint.   D. The glenohumeral joint.

❺ Actually the ankle joint is the joint in which?

A. The distal tibia articulates with the distal fibula.

B. Both the distal tibia and fibula articulate with the talus.

C. The talus articulates with the calcaneus.

D. The calcaneus articulates with the navicular bone.

Answers

❶ D   ❷ A   ❸ B   ❹ A   ❺ B

The Vertebral Column
脊柱

3

There are different numbers of vertebral bones (Figure 3–1) at each level: the cervical–7, the thoracic–12, the lumbar–5, the sacral–5 (fused together), and the coccygeal (also known as the tail bone)–4 (fused together as well). Therefore, there are 33 vertebral bones that stack together or articulate with each other through intervertebral joints between two adjacent vertebral bones to make the vertebral curvature (posture). When a baby is born, he/she may present with two primary vertebral curvatures developed as a fetus: both thoracic and sacral levels curve convexly toward the posterior, called kyphosis. As the baby grows and is gradually able to raise his head (around 3 months old), sit (around 6 months old), or stand (around 9–12 months old), the secondary vertebral curvatures will develop respectively at the cervical and lumbar levels which will have the convex curve anteriorly, called lordosis.

At the cephalic end, the vertebral column at the cervical level connects with the occipital bone of the skull through the atlanto-occipital

脊柱每个节段有不同数量的椎骨（图3–1）：7个颈段、12个胸段、5个腰段、5个骶段（已融合在一起）和4个尾骨（也已融合在一起）。因此，有33块椎骨通过相邻两个椎体之间的关节相互叠加或相互连接，构成了脊柱的曲度（姿势）。当婴儿出生时，他/她会呈现两个初始的胎儿发育时形成的脊椎弯曲：即胸部和骶骨纵向曲线向后凸，称为后凸。当婴儿长大并逐渐能够抬起头时（大约3个月龄）、能坐（大约6个月龄）或能站立（9～12个月龄）时，继发性脊椎弯曲将分别在颈椎（抬头）和腰椎（挺直躯干）发育形成，纵向曲线向前，称为前凸。

在头端，脊柱在颈椎水平通过第一颈椎（寰椎）与枕骨基底

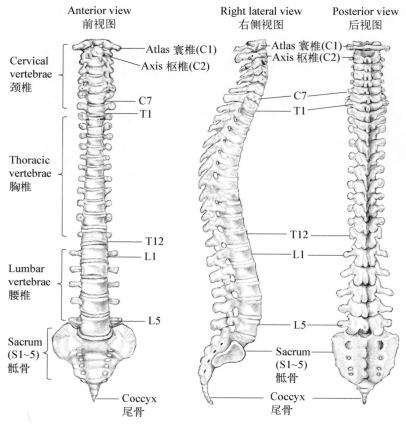

Anterior view
前视图

Right lateral view
右侧视图

Posterior view
后视图

Atlas 寰椎(C1)
Axis 枢椎(C2)

Cervical
vertebrae
颈椎

C7
T1

Thoracic
vertebrae
胸椎

T12
L1

Lumbar
vertebrae
腰椎

L5

Sacrum
(S1~5)
骶骨

Coccyx
尾骨

Figure 3–1　Vertebral Column
（图3-1　脊柱）

joint, located between the base of the skull and first cervical vertebra (the atlas). At the thoracic level, the 12 thoracic vertebrae articulate with 12 pairs of ribs through the costovertebral joints between the rib and the vertebral body, and the costotransverse joints between the ribs and the transverse processes on the thoracic vertebra. Anteriorly these ribs will directly (1st–6th or indirectly (7th–10th) connect with the sternum, with the exception of the 11th and 12th floating ribs. Together, the thoracic vertebra, ribs, and

部之间的寰枕关节相连到颅骨。在胸段,12个胸椎通过与各自对应的肋骨形成肋骨和椎骨体之间的肋椎关节以及肋骨与椎体横突之间形成的肋横突关节而连接在一起。在前部,这些肋骨（第1～6肋）直接或（第7～10肋）间接地与胸骨相连,但不包括第11和第12浮肋。胸椎、肋骨和胸骨共同构成胸腔。

sternum make the chest cavity.

The 5 lumbar vertebrae do not have articulation with other bones except among themselves. They are the most caudal part of the presacral vertebral column (including the lumbar, thoracic, and cervical levels) that hold the trunk of the human body. Due to the location of the lumbar vertebra, it is understood that this level of the spine carries more body weight than other vertebral levels making it an easy target for the occurrence of low back pain.

At the caudal end of the vertebral column, the sacrum, which is a fused bone made up from 5 sacral vertebrae, makes an interlocked connection (the sacroiliac joint) with the ilium bilaterally. The ilium is one of the three hipbones in addition to the pubis and ischium. The hip bone and the sacrum together form the bony wall of the pelvis, which provides the base for the vertebral column as well as the pivot portion for connecting bones of the lower extremity. The coccygeal vertebra is 4-vertebrae fused together, the remnant of the vertebral column, and not functionally important.

Morphologically, each single vertebra includes a large vertebral body, a pair of pedicles and lamina, which surround the vertebral foramen. All of the foramen together form the vertebral canal that contains the spinal canal where the spinal cord rests inside. The single posteriorly-protruded process is the spinous process, while a pair of transverse processes extend from the conjunction between the pedicle and the lamina. Also

5个腰椎除彼此间相关节外，与其他骨无关节连结。它们是控制人体躯干的骶骨以上脊柱（包括腰椎、胸椎和颈椎）最底端的部分。由于位置的原因，腰段脊柱相对于其他阶段会承受更多的体重，从而更容易导致腰痛。

在脊柱尾端，骶骨是由5个骶椎组成的融合骨与双侧髂骨相互连接（骶髂关节）。髂骨是组成髋骨的3块骨头之一，另2块为耻骨和坐骨。髋骨和骶骨共同构成骨盆的骨壁，为脊柱提供基础，也是连接下肢骨的枢轴部分。尾椎由4个椎体融合在一起，是脊柱的残余部分，在功能上不重要。

从形态学上看，每块椎骨包括一个大的椎体、一对椎弓根和一对椎板。这些结构围成椎孔。全部椎孔连接在一起形成骨性椎管，骨性椎管内是含有脊髓的脊髓管，单个向后突出的为棘突，而椎弓根与椎板的结合处向外侧延伸的凸起为一对横突。同时在此结合处，上、下关节突垂直地伸出与邻近椎骨的关节

at this conjunction, superior and inferior articular processes spring out vertically for articulation with the articular processes of the neighboring vertebrae. Each surface of these articular processes is called an articular facet, so the articulation is then called the facet joint. A facet joint is a plane synovial joint that allows gliding and limits segmental spinal movement between two adjoining vertebrae. Besides these two facet joints, the non-synovial intervertebral joint is another joint that pulls two vertebral bodies together with an intervertebral disc between the bodies. These two facet joints and one intervertebral joint work together to allow intervertebral stability as well as mobility.

突形成关节。这些关节突的各个表面被称为小关节面,因此这些关节被称为小关节。小关节是一个平面滑膜关节,可引导和限制节段性脊柱在两个相邻椎体之间的运动。除小关节外,还存在1个通过椎间盘将两相邻椎体连接在一起的非滑膜关节,称为椎体间关节。(两相邻椎骨通过)2个小关节和1个椎间关节一起工作,以保证椎骨间的稳定性和可移动性。

New words

cervical ['sɜːvɪkl] *adj.* 颈的

thoracic [θɔːˈræsɪk] *adj.* 胸椎的

lumbar ['lʌmbə(r)] *adj.* 腰椎的

sacral ['seɪkrəl] *adj.* 骶骨的

coccygeal [kɒkˈsɪdʒɪəl] *adj.* 尾骨的

stack [stæk] *n.* v. 堆叠

articulate [ɑrˈtɪkjulet] *v.* 用关节连接

intervertebral joints 椎间关节

adjacent [əˈdʒeɪsnt] *adj.* 相邻的

curvature ['kɜːvətʃə] *n.* 弯曲

fetus ['fitəs] *n.* 胎儿

kyphosis [kaɪˈfosɪs] *n.* 驼背,脊柱后凸

convexly [kɒnˈvekslɪ] *adv.* 凸面地

lordosis [lɔrˈdosɪs] *n.* 脊柱前凸

cephalic [sɪˈfælɪk] *adj.* 头的,头部的

occipital bone　枕骨

atlantooccipital [æt'læntəʊɒks'ɪpɪtəl] *adj.* 寰枕的

costovertebral [ˌkɔstəu'və:tɪbrəl] *adj.* 肋椎的

costotransverse [kɒstətrænz'vɜ:s] *adj.* 肋（椎骨）横突的

sternum ['stɜ:nəm] *n.* 胸骨

caudal ['kɔdl] *adj.* 尾部的

ilium ['ɪlɪəm] *n.* 髂骨

sacroiliac joint　骶髂关节

pubis ['pju:bɪs] *n.* 耻骨

ischium ['ɪskɪəm] *n.* 坐骨

pivot ['pɪvət] *n.* 枢轴

remnant ['rɛmnənt] *n.* 剩余，遗留

pedicle ['pɛdəkl] *n.* 椎弓根

lamina ['læmənə] *n.* 椎板

morphologically *adv.* 形态学上的

foramen [fəʊ'reɪmən] *n.* 孔

vertebral canal　椎管

posteriorly-protruded　向后突出的

conjunction [kən'dʒʌŋkʃən] *n.* 连接

vertically ['vɜ:tɪklɪ] *adv.* 垂直地

articular facet　关节面（多用于脊柱关节突关节）

adjoining [ə'dʒɔɪnɪŋ] *adj.* 邻接的

Questions

❶ How many vertebral bones in a normal human skeleton?

    A. 29.   B. 31.

    C. 33.   D. 35.

❷ As a baby is able to raise his head up, which one of the curvatures will develop?

    A. The cervical kyphosis.   B. The cervical lordosis.

    C. The lumbar kyphosis.   D. The lumbar lordosis.

❸ Which one of the following bones is not part of the rib cage for making the chest cavity?

A. The thoracic vertebra.　　　　　B. The ribs.

C. The clavicle.　　　　　　　　　D. The sternum.

❹ There are three bones that form the hip bone. What are they?

A. The ilium, the ischium, and the sacrum.

B. The pubis, the ischium, and the sacrum.

C. The ilium, the ischium, and the sacrum.

D. The ilium, the pubis, and the ischium.

❺ The facet joint is actually between _____.

A. two neighboring vertebral bodies

B. two neighboring transverse processes

C. two neighboring articular processes

D. two neighboring spinous processes

Answers

❶ C　　❷ B　　❸ C　　❹ D　　❺ C

Joints and Ligaments
关节和韧带

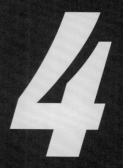

Two adjacent bones join together to make a joint. There are two categories of joints: synovial and non-synovial. Synovial joints (Figure 4–1) are more common in the human body. It is mobile and has a fibrous joint capsule which makes the synovial cavity, a synovial membrane that lines the inner capsule surface, articular cartilage that covers the bone surface, and synovial fluid inside the cavity that lubricates and nourishes the joint. On the other hand, a non-synovial joint is not mobile or nearly immobile. Its bones are united by tight connective tissue without a synovial structure surrounding it.

Synovial joints can further be classified into six different types (Figure 4–2) based on the shape and structure of the joint. 1. The plane joint allows a gliding movement between two flat surfaces (e.g., the acromioclavicular and sternoclavicular joints). 2. The hinge joint acts like a hinge on a door to allow movement in one direction, mostly showing flexion and extension in the sagittal plane (e.g., the elbow,

　　相邻的2块骨组成一个关节。关节分为两类：滑膜关节和非滑膜关节，在人体中滑膜关节（图4-1）更为常见。它具有可动性，有纤维关节囊组成滑膜腔，滑膜覆盖于关节囊内表面，关节软骨覆盖骨面，囊内有滑液起到润滑和滋养关节的作用。另一方面，非滑膜关节由紧密的结缔组织连接，周围没有滑膜结构，其活动性非常小，或几乎不能活动。

　　根据关节的形状和结构，滑膜关节可进一步分为六种不同的关节（图4-2）。① 平面关节，允许关节在2个平面之间滑动（如肩锁关节和胸锁关节）；② 铰链关节，就像门上的铰链，允许关节朝一个方向运动，大多数表现为关节在矢状面上屈曲和伸展（如肘关节、膝关节和踝

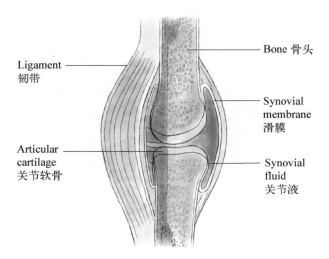

Ligament
韧带

Bone 骨头

Synovial
membrane
滑膜

Articular
cartilage
关节软骨

Synovial
fluid
关节液

Figure 4–1　Synovial joints
（图4–1　滑膜关节）

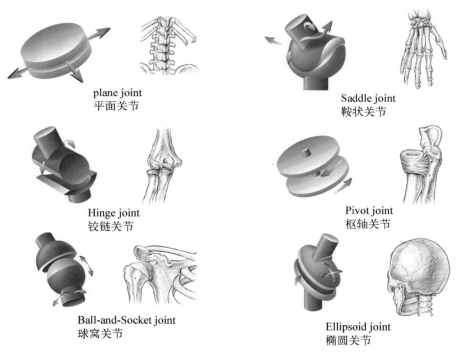

plane joint
平面关节

Saddle joint
鞍状关节

Hinge joint
铰链关节

Pivot joint
枢轴关节

Ball-and-Socket joint
球窝关节

Ellipsoid joint
椭圆关节

Figure 4–2　Synovial joints typing
（图4–2　滑膜关节）

knee, and ankle joints); 3. The pivot joint allows rotatory movement around a single axis in the transverse plane (e.g., the atlantoaxial and proximal and distal radioulnar joints). 4. The condyloid joint uses an ovoid condylar surface to articulate with an elliptical surface to allow movement in the sagittal and coronal planes (e.g., the wrist and metatarsophalangeal joints). 5. The saddle joint allows movements like a rider siting on a saddle moving in the sagittal and coronal planes as well (e.g., the 1st carpometacarpal joint). 6. The ball-and-socket joint is the most mobile joint with a ball-like surface articulating with a socket-like surface to allow movement in all 3-D planes (e.g., the shoulder and hip joints).

Non-synovial joints can be classified as fibrous or cartilaginous based on the type of connective tissue within the articulation. The following three are good examples of fibrous non-synovial joints. 1. A suture, which unites the flat frontal, parietal, temporal, and occipital bones together by thin connective tissue, is often seen in the skull. 2. The gomphosis (the dentoalveolar joints) anchors a tooth into the tooth socket which is stabilized by fibrous tissue. 3. The syndesmosis, seen where the shafts of the radius and ulna (or the shafts of the tibia and fibule) are pulled close to each other, is due to the fibrous interosseous membrane between them. The cartilaginous non-synovial joint can be categorized to be either a symphysis or a synchondrosis. 1. In a symphysis, the bones are joined by fibrocartilage which is in the form of a disk

关节);③ 枢轴关节,允许关节在横断面上绕单轴作旋转运动(例如寰枢关节和桡尺近端、远端关节);④ 髁状关节,由一个卵圆形的髁面与一个椭圆形的凹面相接形成,允许关节在矢状面和冠状面上运动(例如腕关节和掌指关节);⑤ 鞍状关节,指关节之间可以像骑手一样坐在马鞍上,在矢状面和冠状面上移动(例如第1腕掌关节);⑥ 球窝关节,是最灵活的关节,球状表面与套筒状表面连接,允许关节在三维平面内进行运动(如肩关节和髋关节)。

非滑膜关节可根据关节内结缔组织的类型分为纤维性关节和软骨性关节。以下三个是纤维性非滑膜关节的好例子。① 缝合关节,由一个薄薄的结缔组织把平薄的额骨、顶骨、颞部或枕骨连接一起,这种类型的关节往往是在颅骨上看到。② 嵌合关节(牙槽关节),将一颗牙齿由纤维组织稳定在齿槽中。③ 骨间膜连接,如桡骨和尺骨(或胫骨和腓骨)的两骨干通过纤维性骨间膜相互拉拢靠近。软骨性非滑膜关节可以归于骨联合或软骨连合两类。① 在骨联合关节中,骨是由纤维软骨以骨间盘或板的形式连接(例如在2个髋骨之间的耻骨联合和2个椎体之间的椎间盘)。② 在软骨性关节中,骨与透明软骨直接连

or plate (e.g., the symphysis pubis between the two hip bones and the intervertebral disk between two vertebral bodies). 2. In synchondrosis, a bone is directly connected with hyaline cartilage (e.g., the costochondral joints, and the 1st pair of costosternal joint).

Joints are usually reinforced by ligaments that cross over the joint in different planes. A ligament is tight connective tissue with a shape like a cord (e.g., the lateral collateral ligament of the knee) or like a flat band (e.g., the medial collateral ligament of the knee). The main function of a ligament is to stabilize a joint and prevent the joint from injury.

It is worthwhile to note that a synovial joint is mobile in most situations. However, in a certain position, a synovial joint can be immobile or less mobile. This position is kinematically called a close-packed joint. On the other hand, a joint can also be more mobile in a certain position, which is called an open-packed or loose-packed position. In the close-packed position, the two bone surfaces are maximally congruent, and the joint capsule and ligaments are taut resulting in the greatest mechanical stability for the joint. In the open-packed position, the two bone surfaces are minimally congruent, and the joint capsule and ligaments are lax resulting in the least mechanical stability for the joint. Clinically, understanding the structural and mechanical characteristics of a joint may help a clinician better conduct joint mobilization and manipulation techniques.

接（例如肋软骨关节和第一对胸肋关节）。

关节通常是由在不同平面跨过关节的韧带加强。韧带是致密的结缔组织，其形状像一根绳子（例如膝盖的外侧副韧带），或者像扁平的带子（例如膝内侧副韧带）。韧带的主要作用是稳定关节，防止关节损伤。

值得注意的是，在大多数时候，滑膜关节是活动的。然而，在某一位置，滑膜关节是不动的或仅具有很小的可动性，这个位置在关节运动学上称为关节的"锁定"。另一方面，1个关节也可以是在一定的位置时有最大可移动性，这个位置称为"开锁"或松弛位置。在关节锁定位，两个骨表面有最大的契合度，关节囊和韧带处于紧张状态，为关节提供了最大的机械稳定性。在"松弛"位置，两个骨表面有最小的契合度，关节囊和韧带处于松弛状态，为关节提供较小的机械稳定性。临床上，了解关节结构和机械特性可以有助于更好地进行关节松动和相应的手法操作。

New words

adjacent bone 相邻骨

fibrous ['faɪbrəs] *adj.* 纤维性的

synovial [saɪ'novɪəl] *adj.* 滑液的

cartilage ['kɑːtɪlɪdʒ] *n.* 软骨

nourish ['nʌrɪʃ] *v.* 滋养

acromioclavicular [əˌkrəumiəuklə'vikjulə] *adj.* 肩锁的

sternoclavicular [ˌstəːnəuklə'vikjulə] *adj.* 胸锁的

hinge joint 铰链接合

sagittal plane 矢状面

transverse plane 横切面

atlantoaxial [ætlæn'təuksɪəl] *adj.* 寰枢(椎)的

radioulnar joint 桡尺关节

condyloid joint 踝状关节

condylar ['kɒndɪlə(r)] *adj.* 髁的

ovoid ['ovɔɪd] *adj.* 卵形的

elliptical surface 椭圆表面

metatarsophalangeal joint 跖趾关节

saddle joint 鞍形关节

carpometacarpal joint 腕掌关节

ball-and-socket joint 球窝关节

suture ['sutʃə] *n.* 缝合处

frontal bone 额骨

parietal bone 顶骨

temporal bone 颞骨

occipital bone 枕骨

gomphosis [gɒm'fəusɪs] *n.* 嵌合关节

dentoalveolar joint 牙槽关节

syndesmosis [ˌsɪndɛs'məsɪs] *n.* 韧带联合

interosseous membrane 骨间膜

symphysis ['sɪmfəsɪs] *n.* 联合

synchondrosis [ˌsɪŋkɔn'drəusɪs] *n.* 软骨结合

hyaline ['haɪəlɪn] *adj.* 透明的；玻璃似的

costochondral joint　肋软骨连结
costosternal joint　肋胸关节
kinematically [ˌkini'mætik, kai-, -kəl] *adv.* 运动学上的
close-packed joint　闭链关节
open-packed joint　开链关节
congruent ['kɑŋgruənt] *adj.* 契合的

Questions

❶ Which one of the following is not a synovial joint?

A. Between the parietal bone and frontal bone.

B. Between the humerus and the scapula.

C. Between the femur and the tibial plateau.

D. Between the humerus and the radial head.

❷ Which one of the following is a plane joint that allows a gliding movement between two flat bones?

A. The humero glenoid joint.

B. The acromioclavicular joint.

C. The ankle joint.

D. The wrist joint.

❸ Which one of the following is a ball-and-socket joint that allows movement in all 3-D planes?

A. The wrist joint.　　　　　　　　B. The ankle joint.

C. The hip joint.　　　　　　　　　D. The elbow joint.

❹ The left and right hip bones are connected anteriorly through a non-synovial joint, which is called?

A. the syndesmosis　　　　　　　　B. the symphysis

C. the synchondrosis　　　　　　　D. the synovium

⑤ When you stand on your single leg to maintain the stability, you want your knee joint in _____.

A. open-packed position

B. loose-packed position

C. close-packed position

D. All positions above

Answers

❶ A   **❷** B   **❸** C   **❹** B   **❺** C

Anatomical Position and Related Movement Terms
解剖学姿势和相关动作术语

5

In clinical termionology, anatomical position is standing with arms hanging down by the side of the body with palms facing forward. In this position, the front and back of a body or body part are referred to as the anterior (ventral) and the posterior (dorsal) respectively; for instance, there are anterior and posterior interosseous nerves of the forearm. Near the midline and away from the midline are referred to as medial and lateral respectively; for instance, there are medial and lateral collateral ligaments of the elbow and knee. Towards the head and towards the feet are referred to as superior (cranial, cephalic) or inferior (caudal); for instance, there are superior and inferior serratus posterior. On the same or opposite side is referred to as the ipsilateral or the contralateral side; for instance, we may say the ipsilateral lesion verses the contralateral lesion.

Body parts like the head, trunk and extremities move in 3-dimensional planes (Figure 5–1): the sagittal plane is in an anterior-posterior direction, the coronal plane is in a medial-lateral

临床医学术语中,解剖学姿势是指身体直立,上肢垂于躯干两侧,手掌朝向前方。在这种姿势下,身体前方或后方分别被称为前(腹侧)和后(背侧);例如,前臂有前骨间神经和后骨间神经。靠近及远离人体中线分别为内和外,例如肘关节和膝关节分别有内侧和外侧副韧带。靠近头部或足部分别称为上和下(头和尾),例如上下后锯肌。ipsilateral 和 contralateral 分别指同侧和对侧,例如 ipsilateral lesion 指同侧病变,contralateral lesion 指对侧病变。

像头部、躯干和上下肢等身体部位,可在三维平面内进行运动(图5–1):前后方向上的矢状面,左右方向上的冠状面和在解

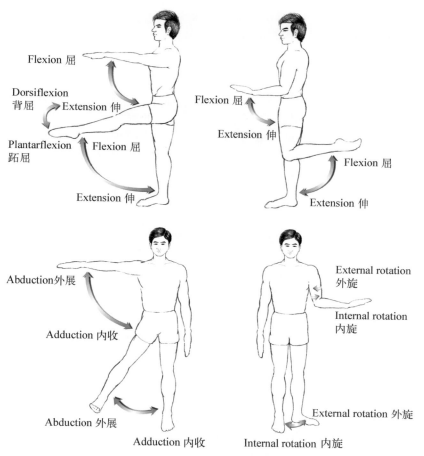

Figure 5–1 3-dimensional planes
（图5–1 三维平面运动）

direction, and the transverse plane is parallel to the floor or ground in the anatomical standing position. In the sagittal plane, movements of body parts in the anterior or posterior direction are referred to as flexion and extension. For example, the head, trunk, upper extremities, and hip move in this plane (most as flexes toward the anterior and extends toward the posterior). However, it should be noted that knee flexion is when the knee bends posteriorly while extension is when

剖学姿势中与地面平行的横断面。在矢状面上肢体前后方向的运动称为屈伸。例如，头部、躯干、上肢以及髋关节可以在这个平面进行运动（多为向前为曲，向后为伸）。然而，需要指出的是，膝关节的屈是指弯曲向后，而伸则指腿部伸直的过程。对于踝关节来说，跖屈是指足前部向下运动，背屈是指足前部向

the knee straightens. For the ankle joint, plantar flexion is when the front part of the foot points down while dorsiflexion is when the front part of the foot pulls upward.

In the coronal plane, body parts move away from (abduct) or move back toward (adduct) the body, e.g., the shoulder and hip movements in this plane. Also, there are a few variations of descriptions for movements in the coronal plane. Lateral flexion is used to describe side bending of the head and trunk; and radial deviation (abduction) and ulnar deviation (adduction) are used for the wrist joint.

In the transverse plane, body parts make rotatory movement by turning left or right. The turning can be referred to as left and right rotations of the head, trunk, and pelvis; internal and external rotations of the shoulder and hip; or pronation and supination of the forearm.

However, due to embryological effects on thumb and ankle development, in the anatomical position, the thumb's (Figure 5–2) flexion and extension occur in the coronal plane, while its abduction and adduction occur in the sagittal plane. Ankle eversion and inversion occur in the coronal plane, while ankle abduction and adduction occur in the transverse plane.

Additionally, the scapula is kind of floating in the coronal plane on the dorsal side of the rib cage. When it slides in a medial-lateral direction, the movements are referred to as protraction (moving away from the thoracic column) or retraction (moving towards the thoracic column). When it slides in the superior-inferior direction, the movements are referred to as elevation

上运动。

在冠状面上,肢体的运动都是偏离(外展)或靠近(内收)躯干,例如肩关节和髋关节的运动可以发生在这个平面。同样,冠状面上的运动描述也有一些特殊性,侧屈用来描述躯干和头部向一侧弯曲,桡偏(外展)和尺偏(内收)用来描述腕部的运动。

在横断面上,身体可以进行向左或向右的旋转运动,旋转的方式有头部和躯干的向前向后旋转,肩关节和髋关节的内旋和外旋,或前臂的旋前和旋后。

然而,因为在拇指和踝关节发育过程中的胚胎学效应,在解剖学姿势中,拇指(图5-2)的屈伸实际上发生在冠状面上,而外展和内收则发生在矢状面上。踝关节外翻和内翻发生在冠状面上,而它的内收和外展则发生在横断面上。

另外,肩胛骨在近似冠状面的胸廓后壁上贴附滑动,当它在内外侧的方向上滑动时,称为前伸(偏离胸段脊柱)和后缩(靠近胸段脊柱)。当它在上下方向滑动时,称为上提(向上运动)或下沉(向下运动)。当肩峰向下外侧旋转时称为内旋,相反的运动

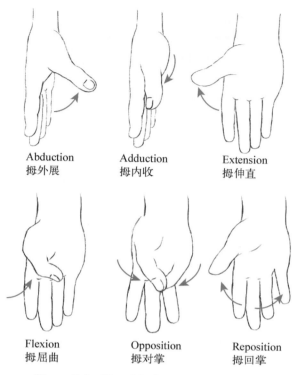

Abduction
拇外展

Adduction
拇内收

Extension
拇伸直

Flexion
拇屈曲

Opposition
拇对掌

Reposition
拇回掌

Figure 5–2   Thumb's flexion and extension
（图5–2   拇指的屈伸）

(superior movement) or depression (inferior movement). When the scapular acromial process rotates laterally and inferiorly, the motion is referred to as scapular downward rotation; while the contrary is referred to as scapular upward rotation.

Opposition and circumduction are two specific joint movements that involve movement in all 3-dimensional planes. Opposition is the typical movement of the thumb by using the thumb tip to touch the tip of all other four fingers. Opposition is very important for pinching actions. Circumduction often happens in the shoulder or hip joint allowing the

称为外旋。

对掌和环转是两种特殊的运动，其可同时发生在三维平面的各个面内。对掌是拇指的一种典型运动，其指拇指分别与其他四个手指相接触，对掌运动对捏拈等动作十分重要。环转动作经常发生在肩关节和髋关节，使远端肢体做出环形动作，而近

distal end of the extremity to make a circular movement, while the proximal end of the extremity remains relatively fixed–looks like a pendulum. Someone with hemiparalysis may demonstrate a circumductory movement during ambulation.

端保持相对固定,整个看起来像一个钟摆。偏瘫患者步行过程中患肢可出现环转运动。

New words

ventral ['vɛntrəl] *adj.* 腹侧的

dorsal ['dɔrsl] *adj.* 背侧的

interosseous nerve　骨间神经

cephalic [sɪ'fælɪk] *adj.* 头的,头部的

caudal ['kɔːdl] *adj.* 尾的,尾部的

serratus [se'reɪtəs] *n.* 锯齿状

plantar flexion [plæntɑː'flekʃn] *n.* 跖曲

dorsiflexion [dɔːsɪ'flekʃən] *n.* 背屈

eversion [ɪ'vɜːʃən] *n.* 外翻

inversion [ɪn'vɜːʃən] *n.* 内翻

deviation [ˌdiːvi'eɪʃn] *n.* 偏离

pronation [prəʊ'neɪʃən] *n.* 旋前

supination [ˌsjuːpɪ'neɪʃən] *n.* 旋后

embryological [ˌembrɪə'lɒdʒɪkl] *adj.* 胚胎学的

protraction [prə'trækʃən] *n.*（肩胛骨）前移（外展）

retraction [rɪ'trækʃn] *n.*（肩胛骨）后移（内收）

scapular acromion　肩胛的肩峰

acromial [ə'krəʊmiəl] *adj.* 肩峰的

circumduction [sɜːkəm'dʌkʃən] *n.* 环行

pinch ['pɪntʃ] *v.* 捏

pendulum ['pendjələm] *n.* 钟摆

hemiparalysis [hemɪpɑː'rələsɪs] *n.* 偏瘫

ipsilateral [ɪpsɪ'lætərəl] *adj.* 同侧的

contralateral [ˌkɒntrə'lætərəl] *adj.* 对侧的

lesion ['liːʒ(ə)n] *n.* 损害

- - - - - - - - - - - - - - - - - - - -(**Questions**)- - - - - - - - - - - - - - - - - - -

❶ A patient is referred to you with a symptom of "muscle spasm of anterior forearm". Where is the body part that the patient gets hurt?

A. The back of the forearm.   B. The front of the forearm.

C. The back of the thigh.   D. The front of the arm.

❷ On a MRI film, a lesion, which causes the contralateral paralysis of upper and lower limbs, is identified at the left brain. Which upper limb or limbs are actually paralyzed?

A. The left upper limb.   B. The right upper limb.

C. Both the left and right limbs.   D. The left lower lower limb.

❸ Standing upright with hands naturally hanging down on either side of your body, you move your right arm away from your body and point to the right side. What is the term can you used to describe the right arm movement?

A. Shoulder flexion.   B. Shoulder adduction.

C. Shoulder abduction.   D. Scapular retraction.

❹ In an anatomical position, when your thumb is away from your body, it is called

_____.

A. thumb abduction   B. thumb adduction

C. thumb extension   D. thumb flexion

❺ The movement that the tip of thumb touches the tip of all other fingers is called

_____.

A. opposition   B. circumduction

C. pronation   D. supination

Answers

❶ D   ❷ B   ❸ C   ❹ A   ❺ A

The Skeletal Muscle System
骨骼肌系统

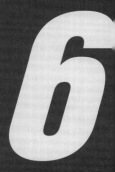

The skeletal muscle system (Figure 6–1) makes up about 40% of the body's mass and their main role is for voluntary movement. Morphologically, there are three types of connective tissue that wraps around the muscle fibers: the endomysium wraps around an individual fiber, the perimysium wraps around a group of muscle fibers, and the epimysium wraps around the entire muscle. These connective tissues work functionally to support, protect, and nourish the muscle fibers.

The individual muscle fiber is the basic unit for muscle contraction. Each of these skeletal muscle fibers is innervated by one alpha motor neuron. Each alpha motor neuron innervates many skeletal muscle fibers. One motor neuron with the muscles it innervates is referred to as a motor unit. Muscles with motor units that contain several hundred muscle fibers (e.g., large muscles of the lower extremity) are designed for gross movement. Muscles with motor units that contain only a few muscle fibers (e.g., extra-ocular muscles of the eye) are

骨骼肌(图6-1)大约占人体总质量的40%,它们的主要任务是完成随意运动。就形态学而言,有三种结缔组织膜包裹在肌纤维周围:包裹单独肌纤维的肌内膜,包裹1束肌纤维的肌束膜,以及包裹整个肌肉的肌外膜。这些结缔组织膜在功能上为肌纤维提供支持、保护和滋养的作用。

单肌纤维是肌肉收缩的基本单位。每一条骨骼肌纤维都由一个α运动神经元支配。每个α运动神经元可支配很多骨骼肌纤维。一个运动神经元加上其所支配的肌纤维被称为一个运动单位。含有的运动单位支配数百条肌纤维的肌肉(如下肢大肌肉)多用于粗大运动,而含有的运动单位仅仅支配几条肌纤维的肌肉(如眼外肌肉)则用于精细运动。

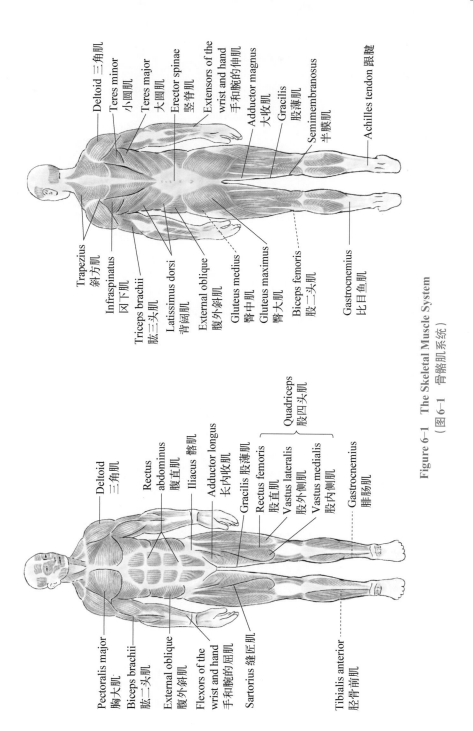

Deltoid 三角肌
Teres minor 小圆肌
Teres major 大圆肌
Erector spinae 竖脊肌
Extensors of the wrist and hand 手和腕的伸肌
Adductor magnus 大收肌
Gracilis 股薄肌
Semimembranosus 半膜肌
Achilles tendon 跟腱

Trapezius 斜方肌
Infraspinatus 冈下肌
Triceps brachii 肱三头肌
Latissimus dorsi 背阔肌
External oblique 腹外斜肌
Gluteus medius 臀中肌
Gluteus maximus 臀大肌
Biceps femoris 股二头肌
Gastrocnemius 比目鱼肌

Deltoid 三角肌
Rectus abdominus 腹直肌
Iliacus 髂肌
Adductor longus 长内收肌
Gracilis 股薄肌
Rectus femoris 股直肌
Vastus lateralis 股外侧肌
Vastus medialis 股内侧肌
Quadriceps 股四头肌
Gastrocnemius 腓肠肌

Pectoralis major 胸大肌
Biceps brachii 肱二头肌
External oblique 腹外斜肌
Flexors of the wrist and hand 手和腕的屈肌
Sartorius 缝匠肌
Tibialis anterior 胫骨前肌

Figure 6-1 The Skeletal Muscle System
（图 6-1 骨骼肌系统）

designed for fine motor control.

A muscle can cross one joint as a single-joint muscle or cross two or more joints as a two- or multi-joint muscle, depending on where the muscle's proximal (origin) and distal (insertion) attachments are on the bones. By putting the origin and insertion of a muscle into a 3-D space, we will be able to understand that the muscle can move a joint in the sagittal, coronal, and/or transverse planes. For example, the biceps brachii muscle has its origins on the supraglenoid tubercle (for its long head) and the coronoid process of the scapula (for its short head), and its insertion on the radial tuberosity of the radius. Because of its origins and insertion, this muscle is able to flex the elbow in the sagittal plane and supinate the forearm in the transverse plane. Therefore, during manual muscle testing (MMT), the strength of the biceps brachii can be properly tested by asking your subject to flex the elbow and supinate the forearm.

The direction and strength of a joint movement depends on the vector of forces made by the group of muscles surrounding the joint. For example, elbow flexion depends on the action of the biceps brachii, brachialis, pronator teres and brachioradialis.

Further, there are three types of muscle contractions often used for exercise. First, in an isometric contraction, the muscle contracts but remains in place without changing its length. The examples would be holding a basket on your forearm without moving it,or pushing or pulling an object that is immovable.

1块肌肉是跨过1个关节成为单关节肌还是跨过两个或多个关节成为双关节肌或多关节肌取决于肌肉的近端(起点)和远端(止点)在骨骼上附着点位置。通过把肌肉的起点和止点投放到三维空间中,我们可以了解肌肉在矢状面、冠状面或横断面上对关节运动的作用。例如,肱二头肌的起点在盂上结节(长头)和肩胛骨的喙突(短头),止点在桡骨的桡骨粗隆。由于其起点和止点的位置,这块肌肉可以在矢状面上屈肘关节及在水平面上后旋前臂。所以,徒手肌力测试(MMT)时,可以通过让受试者嘱其屈肘关节和后旋前臂来检查肱二头肌的肌力。

关节活动的方向和力量取决于关节周围所包绕的肌肉产生的力量矢量。例如,肘关节屈曲取决于肱二头肌、肱肌、旋前圆肌和肱桡肌的共同作用。

进一步而言,人体运动中存在三种肌肉收缩形式。第一种,等长收缩,肌肉收缩但长度维持不变,例如当你用前臂挎着一个篮子但并没有移动它,或推或拉一个不能移动的物体时的用力情况;第二种,等张收缩,当肌肉

Second, in an isotonic contraction, the muscle contracts to shorten with the same tension. Isotonic contractions can be further classified into concentric and eccentric contractions. A concentric contraction is when a muscle shortens as it contracts, while an eccentric contraction is when the muscle lengthens slowly as it still keeps contraction. These two isotonic contractions can be identified as an example when a person is performing a biceps curl exercise with a 2-kg dumbell weight in his hand. When one bends the elbow to pull the dumbbell up towards the shoulder he is performing a concentric contraction of the biceps brachii muscle. When the dumbbell is lowered by slowly extending the elbow, an eccentric contraction of the muscle is performed. The third type of contraction is an isokinetic contraction in which the muscle contracts similarly to an isotonic contraction but at a constant speed. Usually, a device called an isokinetic dynamometer is needed to perform and measure the isokinetic contraction.

Muscles are often protected by accessory structures that prevent exposure to potential injury. A bursa is a synovial membrane-like closed sac that contains synovial fluid to minimize friction as a tendon slides over a bone during a muscle movement (e.g., the subacromial bursa protects the supraspinatus muscle). A synovial sheath is also a synovial-membrane-like tube structure that wraps around tendons to decrease friction between the muscle tendons and surrounding

缩短时,肌肉张力相同。等张收缩可以进一步被分为向心收缩和离心收缩。向心收缩的定义是肌肉收缩时其长度缩短,而离心收缩与向心收缩相反,其定义是在肌肉长度逐渐增加时,其仍在收缩状态。这两种等张收缩方式可以通过手持2千克哑铃做肱二头肌屈曲运动的例子来加以区分。当曲肘关节把手中的哑铃拉向肩部时,肱二头肌做的是向心收缩;当伸肘缓慢放下哑铃时,肱二头肌进行的是离心收缩;第三种,等速收缩,此收缩形式类似于等长收缩,但是其速度维持恒定。通常情况下,需要一种叫作等速训练仪(测力计)的装置来进行等速收缩训练及肌力测试。

肌肉通常会通过辅助结构来保护其免受到潜在损伤。滑囊是一种滑膜样闭合囊,含有滑液,可以最大限度地减少肌肉活动时肌腱在骨骼上滑动时的摩擦(例如,肩峰下滑囊用于保护冈上肌)。滑膜鞘也是一种滑膜样的管状结构包绕在肌腱周围用于减少肌腱和周围组织之间的摩擦,这些结构常见于跨过腕关节和踝关节的长肌肉。肌内

structures. They are mostly found in long muscles that cross wrist and ankle joints. An intramuscular septum is the lamina of deep fascia that separate and sometimes surround muscle groups (e.g., the muscle septum that separates the leg muscles into anterior, lateral, and posterior groups). They are often continuous with periosteum. A retinaculum is a thickening of deep fascia that serves to hold tendons close to bones as a joint is moving and some muscles around the joint are contracting (e.g., the flexor retinaculum over the carpal tunnel keeps the wrist flexor muscles from bowstringing).

隔膜是用于分隔或包裹在一组肌群周围的深筋膜（例如，肌肉隔膜将腿部肌肉分为前、中、后群），它们经常与骨膜相连。支持带是深筋膜的增厚，其用于当关节活动肌肉收缩时，使肌腱贴近骨面滑动（例如，腕管上的屈肌支持带可避免腕屈肌弓形膨出）。

New words

skeletal ['skɛlətl] *adj.* 骨骼的
morphologically [mɔːfə'lɒdʒɪklɪ] *adv.* 形态学
connective tissue [kə'nɛktɪv'tɪʃu] *n.* 结缔组织
endomysium [endə'mɪzɪəm] *n.* 肌内膜
perimysium [pɛrɪ'mɪzɪəm] *n.* 肌束膜
epimysium [epɪ'mɪsɪəm] *n.* 肌外膜
contraction [kən'trækʃn] *n.* 收缩
innervate [ɪ'nɜːveɪt] *vt.* 使……受神经支配
alpha motor neuron α 运动神经元
gross movement 粗大运动
extraocular [ɛkstrə'ɑkjələ] *adj.* 眼外的
multi-joint muscle 跨多关节肌
origin ['ɒrɪdʒɪn] *n.* 起点
insertion [ɪn'sɜːʃ(ə)n] *n.* 止点
sagittal ['sædʒətəl] *adj.* 矢状的
coronal [kə'rəʊnəl] *adj.* 冠状的
transverse planes 横断面

biceps brachii muscle　肱二头肌

supraglenoid tubercle　盂上结节

coronoid process　*n.* 喙突

scapula ['skæpjʊlə]　*n.* 肩胛骨

radial tuberosity　桡骨粗隆

radius ['redɪəs]　*n.* 桡骨

supinate ['sʊpənet]　*vt.* 旋后

vector ['vɛktə]　*n.* 矢量

brachialis [b'reɪkjəlɪs]　*n.* 肱肌

pronator teres　旋前圆肌

brachioradialis [breɪkɪəreɪdɪ'eɪlɪs]　*n.* 肱桡肌

isometric contraction　等长收缩

isotonic contraction　等张收缩

concentric and eccentric contractions　向心和离心收缩

isokinetic ['aɪsəukɪ'netɪk]　*adj.* 等速；等动力的

isokinetic dynamometer　等速测力计

bursa ['bɜːsə]　*n.* 囊，滑囊

synovial membrane-like　滑膜样

friction ['frɪkʃən]　*n.* 摩擦

subacromial [sʌ'bækrəmɪəl]　*adj.* 肩峰下的

supraspinatus muscle　冈上肌

synovial sheath　滑膜鞘

intramuscular septum　肌内隔膜

deep fascia　深筋膜

periosteum [pɛrɪ'ɑstɪəm]　*n.* 骨膜

retinaculum [rɛtə'nækjələm]　*n.* 支持带

------------------------------ ◀ **Questions** ▶ ------------------------------

❶ The connective tissue that wraps around a group of muscle fibers within a muscle is _____.

    A. the endomysium　　　　　　　　　B. the perimysium

C. the epimysium   D. the periosteum

❷ Which one of the following is correct description of a motor unit?

A. One alpha motor neuron innervates many skeletal muscle fibers.

B. One alpha motor neuron innervates one skeletal muscle fiber.

C. One gamma motor neuron innervates one skeletal muscle fiber.

D. Many alpha motor neurons innervate one skeletal muscle.

❸ In a 3-D space in an anatomical position, the biceps brachii muscle is able to perform elbow flexion and forearm supination in _____ planes.

A. sagittal and transverse   B. sagittal and coronal

C. coronal and transverse   D. sagittal only

❹ You are asked to bend your right elbow and hold a 3 kilograms weight in your hand without moving at all. What exercise are you practicing for your right biceps brachii muscle?

A. Concentric contraction.   B. Eccentric contraction.

C. Isometric contraction.   D. Isokinetic contraction.

❺ As a tight connective tissue, the structure that is often seen to stabilize the tendon or tendons of long muscles in place at a joint area is _____.

A. the ligament   B. the retinaculum

C. the bursa   D. the synovial membrane

Answers

❶ B   ❷ A   ❸ A   ❹ C   ❺ D

The Central Nervous System
中枢神经系统

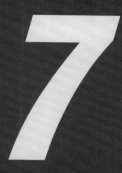

The human nervous system consists of the central and the peripheral nervous systems (Figure 7–1). The nerve cell, or the neuron is the basic functional unit of the system. The components of each neuron consist of a cell body, an axon, and dendrites. Neurons are connected through synapses, which are structures that pass neural signals. The central nervous system (Figure 7–1), including the brain and spinal cord, is wrapped by meninges in the cranial cavity for the brain and in the spinal canal for the spinal cord. The cranial cavity and spinal canal, both filled with cerebral fluid in which the brain and spinal cord float in, communicate through the foramen magnum.

The human brain acts as the headquarter or the command center for the body by receiving input from the sensory organs for information integration and then sending outputs to the muscles for task-oriented movements. The brain weighs about 1.5 kilograms which is about 2% of total body weight. There are over 100 billion neurons in

神经系统由中枢神经系统和周围神经系统组成(图7–1)。神经系统的基本功能单位是神经细胞,也叫神经元。每个神经元都有细胞体、轴突和树突。神经元通过传递神经信号的突触连接。中枢神经系统(图7–1)包括脑和脊髓,脑被脑膜包裹在颅腔内,而脊髓则被脑脊膜包裹在脊髓(椎)管内。颅腔和脊髓(椎)管通过枕骨大孔相通,里面充满了脑脊液及浮在脑脊液里的脑和脊髓。

大脑是我们身体的指挥或控制中心,它可以接收由感觉器官输入的信息进行整合,然后将信息输出给相关肌肉,从而完成任务导向的相关运动。脑重约1.5千克,约占整个体重的2%。大脑中大约有860亿个神经元,由端脑、脑干和小脑组成,其中

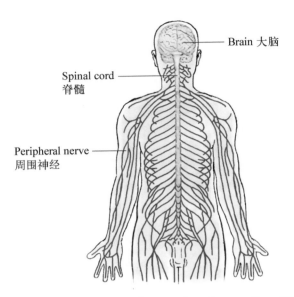

Figure 7-1　The Central Nervous System–the yellow portion of the figure, including the brain and spinal cord

（图7-1　中枢神经系统—图中黄色的部分，包括脑和脊髓）

the human brain which make up the cerebrum, brainstem, and cerebellum, with the cerebrum being the largest. The cerebrum includes the left and right hemispheres. The brainstem is immediately underneath the cerebrum and the cerebellum sits on the dorsal side of the brainstem.

The outer layer of the cerebral hemisphere is the cerebral cortex which is composed of wrinkled structures known as gyri. Gyri are gray matter of the cerebrum and made up by neurons. The fissure between two gyri is called a sulcus. Underneath the cerebral cortex is the white matter that is made up by nerve fibers connecting neurons. Functionally, the left hemisphere is responsible for language, logical thinking, analytical and/or mathematic activities; while the right hemisphere is

端脑是最大的。端脑分为左半球和右半球，脑干位于端脑正下面，小脑位于脑干的背面。

大脑半球的外层是大脑皮质，由褶皱结构组成，这些结构被称为脑回，是由神经元胞体构成的大脑灰质。两脑回之间的裂缝称为脑沟。在大脑皮质的下方是由神经元的神经纤维构成的白质。从功能上讲，左半球负责的是语言、逻辑思维、分析和/或数学活动；而右半球负责的是艺术和音乐活动及空间定位。

responsible for artistic and musical activities, as well as spatial orientation.

The cerebral cortex consists of four lobes (frontal, parietal, temporal, and occipital) that are separated by fissures or sulci. The frontal lobe, located at the front of the brain, is involved in motor function, personality, and language (the left side). The parietal lobe, just posterior to the frontal lobe but superior to the temporal lobe, is mainly responsible for sensory information processing and integration (including proprioception). The temporal lobe, inferior to the parietal lobe, is responsible for memory, hearing processing, and language recognition. The occipital lobe, posterior to the parietal and temporal lobes, is mainly the primary visual cortex.

Hidden inside the cerebrum are the limbic system and the basal ganglia. The limbic system is formed by a group of brain structures and located on the medial border of the hemisphere and is responsible for functions related to emotion, motivation, behavior, and memory. The basal ganglia are also formed by a group of nuclei which are deep within the cerebral hemisphere and are primarily for processing motor-control related information.

The brainstem consists of (from rostral to caudal) the midbrain, pons, and medulla. The midbrain processes information for eye ball movement, visual, and hearing information. The pons is the key structure bridging the cerebrum and the cerebellum and is also functionally for eye ball movement, as well as facial sensory and motor signals, hearing, balance, and even

大脑皮质由四个脑叶组成（额叶、顶叶、颞叶和枕叶），由裂沟或脑沟分开。额叶位于大脑前部，包括运动功能、性格甚至语言（左半球）。顶叶位于额叶后面，颞叶上方，主要用于感觉信息（包括本体感觉）的处理和整合。颞叶，位于顶叶下方，用于记忆、听觉处理和语言识别。枕叶，位于顶叶和颞叶的后部，主要是视觉皮质的位置。

大脑内隐藏的是边缘叶系统和基底神经节。边缘叶由一组大脑结构构成，位于大脑半球的内侧边缘，负责处理与情绪、动机、行为和记忆有关的功能。基底神经节也是由位于大脑半球深处的一组神经核团组成的，主要用于处理运动控制相关的信息。

脑干由（从上到下）中脑、脑桥和延髓组成。中脑负责处理眼球运动、视觉以及听觉的信息。脑桥是连接大脑和小脑的关键结构，也参与眼动、面部感觉和运动、听觉、平衡甚至呼吸的功能。延髓是脑干的最末端，是内脏器官活动的调节中枢，如

breathing. The medulla, the most caudal part of the brainstem, is the center that regulates internal organ activities like breathing, heart beating, and digestion. So, the medulla can be sometimes called "the life center".

The cerebellum is located posterior to the pons and medulla. Its major role is to process and integrate motor-sensory (proprioceptive) signals from the body. Proper cerebellar function will ensure proper muscle tone, equilibrium, and coordinated movements during daily tasks.

The spinal cord is continuous with the medulla as a long and cylindrical structure from the foramen magnum to the 2nd lumbar vertebral level. In a transverse section, the centrally-located butterfly-like structure is the gray matter and the surrounding structure is the white matter. These gray and white matters receive and process information from higher level neurons and/or peripheral neural receptors and then project the processed signals out to higher level neurons or to the muscles in the body. There are 31 segments for the spinal cord including 8 cervical, 12 thoracic, 5 lumbar, 5 sacral, and 1 coccygeal. These 31 segments send out 31 pairs of spinal nerves to target areas or structures throughout the whole body.

呼吸、心跳和消化。所以，延髓有时被称为"生命中心"。

小脑位于脑桥和延髓的后面，它的主要作用是处理和整合来自身体的运动—感觉（本体感觉）信号。完整的小脑功能将保证日常生活任务中合适的肌肉张力、平衡和协调的运动。

脊髓是一个从枕骨大孔延伸到第二腰椎水平的长圆柱状结构。在其横断面上，位于中心位置的蝴蝶状结构是灰质，周围结构是白质。这些灰质和白质接收和处理来自较高级神经元和/或周围神经感受器的信息，然后将处理过的信号投射到较高级别的神经元或肌肉。脊髓有31个节段，包括颈段8个，胸段12个，腰段5个，骶段5个，尾段1个。这31个节段发出31对脊神经至全身各个目标区域或结构。

New words

peripheral nervous system　周围神经系统
axon ['æksɑn] *n.* 轴突
dendrite ['dendraɪt] *n.* 树突

synapse ['saɪnæps] *n.* 突触

meninges [mɪ'nɪndʒiːz] *n.* 脑膜

cranial cavity 颅腔

cerebral fluid 脑脊液

foramen magnum 枕骨大孔

sensory organs 感觉器官

integration [ˌɪntɪ'greɪʃn] *n.* 整合

cerebrum [sə'rɪbrəm] *n.* 大脑

brainstem ['brenstɛm] *n.* 脑干

cerebellum ['sɛrə'bɛləm] *n.* 小脑

cerebral cortex ['serəbrəl'kɔː(r)teks] 大脑皮质

gyri ['dʒaɪərаɪ] *n.* 脑回

gray matter [grei 'mætə] *n.* 灰质

fissure ['fɪʃə(r)] *n.* 裂缝

sulcus ['sʌlkəs] *n.* 脑沟

spatial orientation 空间定位

lobe [ləʊb] *n.* 脑叶

frontal lobe ['frʌntlləʊb] *n.* 额叶

parietal lobe [pə'raɪətəlləʊb] *n.* 顶叶

temporal lobe ['tempərəlləʊb] *n.* 颞叶

occipital lobe [ɔk'sɪpɪtlləʊb] *n.* 枕叶

integration ['ɪntə'greʃən] *n.* 集成；综合

proprioception [ˌproprɪə'sɛpʃən] *n.* 本体感受

caudal ['kɔdl] *adj.* 尾部的，近尾部的

limbic system 边缘系统

basal ganglia 基底神经节

nuclei ['njʊklɪˌaɪ] *n.* 核（复数）

midbrain ['mɪdbreɪn] *n.* 中脑

pons [pɑnz] *n.* 脑桥

medulla [mɪ'dʌlə] *n.* 延髓

equilibrium [ˌikwɪ'lɪbrɪəm] *n.* 平静

coordinated movements 协调运动

foramen magnum 枕骨大孔

cylindrical [sə'lɪndrɪkl] *adj.* 圆柱形的；圆柱体的
transverse section [træns'vɜːs'sekʃən] *n.* 横切面；横断面
coccygeal [kɑk'sɪdʒɪəl] *adj.* 尾骨的

Questions

1 Which one of the following structures is considered to be the central nervous system?

A. The brain and cranial nerves.　　　B. The brain and the spinal cord.

C. The spinal cord only.　　　D. The brain only.

2 In term of location, the cerebellum is immediately _____.

A. anterior to the cerebrum　　　B. posterior to the cerebrum

C. anterior to the brainstem　　　D. posterior to the brainstem

3 A patient with traumatic brain injury to the right hemisphere, which one of the following dysfunction might be identified?

A. Language.　　　B. Spatial orientation.

C. Logical thinking.　　　D. Analytical skills.

4 One of your patients with injury to his occipital lobe may demonstrate to you _____.

A. visual deficit　　　B. hearing deficit

C. personality change　　　D. memory decrease

5 The center that regulates internal organ activities like breathing, heart beating, and digestion is located at _____.

A. the cerebellum　　　B. the midbrain

C. the pons　　　D. the medulla

Answers

1 B　　**2** D　　**3** B　　**4** A　　**5** D

The Peripheral Nervous System
周围神经系统

8

The peripheral nervous system (PNS) (Figure 8–1) acts as the relay station between the central nervous system (CNS) and the body by transmitting sensory information to the CNS and motor signals to target body areas or structures. The PNS consists of 12 pairs of cranial nerves and their ganglia if available, 31 pairs of spinal nerves, 31 pairs of dorsal root ganglia, and the autonomic nervous system. Ganglia are aggregations of neuronal cell bodies outside the CNS and can be sensory or motor. Neurons in the sensory ganglia, such as dorsal root ganglia (DRG) of the spinal nerve and trigeminal ganglia of the trigeminal nerve are neurons processing sensory signals preliminarily before the signals can be sent into the CNS for further processing. The motor ganglia contain neurons of the autonomic system (including sympathetic and parasympathetic systems) that receive input from the CNS and send out motor signals for activities of internal organs.

周围神经系统(PNS)(图8-1)作为中枢神经系统(CNS)与机体之间的中继站,通过向中枢神经系统传递感觉信息,并将运动信号传递给目标部位或结构。周围神经系统包括12对脑神经及其神经节、31对脊神经、31对背根神经节和自主神经系统。神经节是中枢神经系统外神经细胞的聚集体,可以是感觉或运动神经元。像脊神经的背根神经节(DRG)和三叉神经的三叉神经节内的神经元,在信号送入中枢神经系统进行进一步处理之前,会对接收到的感觉信息进行初级处理。运动神经节含有自主神经系统(包括交感和副交感系统)的神经元,接受中枢神经系统的输入,并发出运动信号,用于内脏活动。

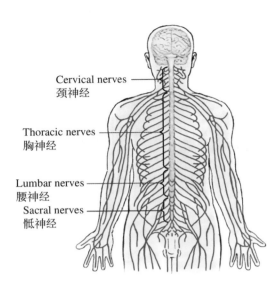

Cervical nerves
颈神经

Thoracic nerves
胸神经

Lumbar nerves
腰神经

Sacral nerves
骶神经

Figure 8-1   The peripheral nervous system (those blue lines in the figure). There are no cranial nerves, sympathetic and parasympathetic nerves drawn here
（图8-1   外周神经系统—图中蓝色线条部分。这里12对脑神经，交感和副交感神经没有绘出）

Cranial nerves 1 to 12 (CN Ⅰ to CN Ⅻ) are kind of like the spinal nerves that are paired for each of them and functionally similar. Some of them carry special sensory information to the brain such as smell (CN Ⅰ – the olfactory nerve), vision (CN Ⅱ – the optical nerve), taste (parts of CN Ⅶ and Ⅸ –the facial and glossopharyngeal nerves), and hearing (the cochlear portion of CN Ⅷ – the vestibulocochlear nerve). A few of them carry motor impulses out for eye movement (CN Ⅲ, Ⅳ, and Ⅵ –the oculomotor, trochlear, and abducens nerves), jaw movement (the 3rd branch of CN Ⅴ –the trigeminal nerve), facial expression (CN Ⅶ –the facial nerve), swallowing and speaking (CN Ⅸ and Ⅹ –the glossopharyngeal and vagus nerves), and tongue movement (CN Ⅻ –the hypoglossal

第1～12脑神经（CN Ⅰ至 CN Ⅻ）类似于脊神经，成对存在，功能相似。它们中的一些将特殊感觉信息传递给脑，如嗅觉（CN Ⅰ—嗅觉神经）、视觉（CN Ⅱ—视神经）、味觉（CN Ⅶ和CN Ⅸ的一部分—面部和舌咽神经）、听觉（CN Ⅷ的耳蜗部分—前庭蜗神经）和平衡觉（CN Ⅷ的前庭神经）。其他脑神经会携带运动信号用于眼球运动（CN Ⅲ、Ⅳ和Ⅵ—动眼神经、滑车神经和外展神经）、下颌骨运动（CN Ⅴ-3—三叉神经的第三支）、面部表情（CN Ⅶ—面神经）、吞咽和说话（CN Ⅸ和Ⅹ—舌咽神经和迷走神经）以及舌运动（CN Ⅻ—舌下神经）。此外四条脑神经

nerve). Also 4 of these cranial nerves (CNs Ⅲ, Ⅶ, Ⅸ, Ⅹ) may carry parasympathetic signals out to targeted glands and internal organs.

Each of the 31 pairs of spinal nerves (sometimes named the spinal roots)(Figure 8-1) contain both afferent sensory fibers from the dorsal root ganglia to the CNS and efferent motor fibers from the spinal cord to targeted muscles. The individual spinal nerve exits the vertebral canal through the intervertebral foramen to innervate the body in a pattern of nerve distribution that corresponds to the spinal segment. Such a pattern is called a dermatome (sensory) or a myotome (motor) in terms of sensory or motor innervations. For instance, the 6th cervical spinal nerve (C6) has its dermatome (the afferent informtion) for the thumb and its myotome (the efferent information) for elbow flexion. Thus, tingling and numbness around the thumb (both the dorsal and palmar sides), and/or a deficit of elbow flexion could be one of the indications for a C6 problem. Further, after the intervertebral foramen, fibers of a spinal nerve (root) will bundle with fibers from one or more spinal nerves (roots) to make one or more peripheral nerves. For example, some C6 fibers will be bundled with some C5 fibers to make the musculocutaneous nerve or with some C5 and C7 fibers to make the long thoracic nerve, or with C5, C7, and T1 fibers to make the median nerve.

The autonomic nervous system is comprised of the sympathetic and parasympathetic nervous systems (SNS and PSNS). Centrally, the SNS

（CN Ⅲ、Ⅶ、Ⅸ、Ⅹ）也可传导副交感神经信号至靶腺体和内脏。

31对脊神经（有时称为脊神经根）（图8-1）中的每一根都含有从背根神经节到中枢神经系统的传入感觉神经纤维和从脊髓到目标肌肉的传出运动神经纤维。每对由椎管通过椎间孔发出的脊神经，对身体支配的神经分布模式是与脊髓节段相对应的。根据感觉或运动神经支配，这种模式被称为皮节（感觉）（Dermatome）或肌节（运动）（Myotome）。例如，C6对应的有拇指的皮节（感觉传入）和屈肘的肌节（运动传出）。因此，拇指周围的刺痛和麻木（包括背侧和掌侧）和/或肘关节屈曲功能不足可能是C6问题的指征之一。此外，出椎间孔后，脊神经（根）的纤维将与一个或多个脊髓神经（根）的纤维结合成束，形成一个或多个周围神经。例如，C6的一些纤维将与一些C5纤维汇合成一束为肌皮神经，或与C5和C7的一些纤维合股形成胸长神经，或与C5、C7和T1纤维形成正中神经。

自主神经系统由交感神经（SNS）和副交感神经系统（PSNS）组成。在中枢神经系统中，交感

neurons are located in the T1–L2 spinal segments and send out their sympathetic fibers to join the spinal nerves from the same segment and to synapse with neurons in the peripheral SNS motor ganglia along the vertebral column. The neurons of the PSNS are in the brainstem and S2–4 spinal segments. These neurons send out their parasympathetic fibers as the vagus nerve and part of S2–4 spinal nerves to synapse with neurons in the peripheral PSNS ganglia on the surfaces of target organs. These peripherally located SNS and PSNS neurons innervate targeted internal organs consequently controlling and regulating them in a coordinated way. Functionally, the sympathetic nervous system is responsible for “fight and flight” activities–think about running in an 800-meter race (sympathetic excitation); while the parasympathetic system is the opposite by controlling “rest and digest” things–think about when you are sleeping (parasympathetic excitation).

神经元位于脊髓T1～L2节段，并发出交感神经纤维混入同一节段的脊神经，并与脊柱周围交感运动神经节内的神经元形成突触。副交感神经的神经元位于脑干和脊髓S2～4节段，这些神经元发出的副交感神经纤维构成迷走神经和S2～4脊神经的一部分，在靶器官表面的副交感神经节内与周围神经元形成突触。这些外周交感和副交感神经，相互协调并有次序地支配和管理靶器官。在功能上，交感神经系统负责“拼斗和奔跑”类的活动——想想在800米赛跑中跑步的时候；而副交感神经系统则相反，控制“休息和消化”类的活动——想想你睡觉的时候。

New words

cranial nerves　脑神经
ganglia ['gæŋglɪə] *n.* 神经节
dorsal root ganglia　背根神经节
autonomic nervous system　自主神经系统
aggregation [ˌægrɪ'geɪʃn] *n.* 聚集
trigeminal nerve [traɪ'dʒemɪnlnəːv] *n.* 三叉神经
sympathetic and parasympathetic　交感和副交感
olfactory nerve [ɔl'fæktəriː nəːv] *n.* 嗅觉神经

optical nerve ['ɒptɪkəlnə:v] *n.* 视神经

cochlear ['kɒklɪə] *adj.* 耳蜗的

vestibulocochlear nerve ['vestɪbjʊləʊkəʊklɪəərnə:v] *n.* 前庭蜗神经

oculomotor nerve [ˌɒkjʊlə'məʊtənə:v] *n.* 动眼神经

trochlear nerve ['trɒklɪənə:v] *n.* 滑车神经

abducens nerve [æb'dju:sənznə:v] *n.* 外展神经

swallowing [s'wɒləʊɪŋ] *n.* 吞咽

glossopharyngeal nerve [ˌglɑsofə'rɪndʒɪəlnə:v] *n.* 舌咽神经

vagus nerve ['veɪgəsnə:v] *n.* 迷走神经

hypoglossal nerve [ˌhaɪpə'glɒsəlnə:v] *n.* 舌下神经

gland [glænd] *n.* 腺体

vertebral canal ['və:tibrəlkə'næl] *n.* 椎管

intervertebral foramen [intə'və:tɪbrəlfə'reɪmen] *n.* 椎间孔

spinal segment ['spaɪnəl'segmənt] *n.* 脊髓节段

dermatome ['dɜ:mətəʊm] *n.* 皮节

myotome ['maɪəˌtom] *n.* 肌节

tingling ['tɪŋgl] *n.* 刺痛

dorsal and palmar sides 背侧和掌侧

musculocutaneous nerve [ˌmʌskjʊləʊkjʊ'teɪnɪəsnə:v] *n.* 肌皮神经

long thoracic nerve 胸长神经

median nerve ['mi:di:ənnə:v] *n.* 正中神经

synapse [sɪ'næps] *n.* 突触

Questions

❶ Normally, how many pairs of spinal nerves are in a human body?

    A. 29.   B. 31.

    C. 33.   D. 35.

❷ Based on the definition described in the text, the motor ganglia _____

    A. are the aggregation of neuronal cell bodies inside the CNS.

    B. are the aggregation of neuronal cell bodies inside muscles.

C. contain neurons processing sensory signals before the signals can be sent into the CNS for further processing.

D. contain neurons of autonomic system that receive input from the CNS and send out motor signals for activities of internal organs.

❸ The 8th cranial nerve, the vestibulocochlear nerve, is responsible for sensory of _____.

A. balance and hearing   B. balance and smelling

C. hearing and vision   D. vision and tasting

❹ The following sentence: "The individual spinal nerve exits out the vertebral canal through the intervertebral foramen to innervate the body in a pattern of sensor", is actually the description of _____.

A. dermatome   B. myotome

C. a peripheral cutaneous nerve   D. a peripheral motor nerve

❺ The sympathetic nervous system is usually located in the _____.

A. C1–7 spinal segments   B. T1–L2 spinal segments

C. L3–S1 spinal segments   D. S2–4 spinal segments

Answers

❶ B   ❷ D   ❸ A   ❹ D   ❺ B

The Chest Cavity and Its Contents
胸腔及其内容

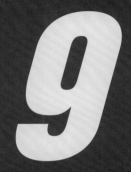

The chest cavity (Figure 9–1) is a hollow space surrounded by the sternum, the ribs, and thoracic vertebral column, and is separated from the abdominal cavity by the diaphragm. The chest cavity contains two lungs on either side, with the heart, trachea, esophagus, and large vessels between the lungs (Figure 9–2). Both left and right lungs are wrapped by the double-layered pleura.

A person's heart is normally about the size of their fist and has four chambers: left and right atria and ventricles. It sits on top of the central and leftward surface of the diaphragm and acts like an engine, receiving blood to the atria and pumping it out through the ventricles. The oxygenated blood is from the lungs to the left atrium. The left ventricle receives oxygenated blood from the left atrium and then pumps it to the whole body through the aorta. Deoxygenated blood returns back to the right atrium to complete the systematic circulation. The right ventricle receives deoxygenated blood from the right atrium

胸腔（图9–1）是由胸骨、肋骨和胸椎围成的中空的腔体，并通过膈肌与腹腔分隔。两肺位于胸腔的两侧，心脏、气管、食管和大血管位于两肺之间（图9–2）。左肺和右肺均由双层的胸膜包裹。

一个人的心脏一般和本人的拳头大小相当，有4个腔：左、右心房和心室。心位于膈肌的中央偏左侧，就像一台发动机，通过心房接收血液并通过心室泵出血液。含氧血从肺部到左心房，左心室从左心房获得含氧血并将其通过主动脉泵向全身，然后脱氧血液返回右心房完成体循环。右心室接收来自右心房的脱氧血液，然后通过肺动脉将其泵入肺部，以供肺部的二氧化碳与氧气的交换。完成交换后，新鲜含氧的血液将通过肺静脉回流到左心房，完成肺循环。

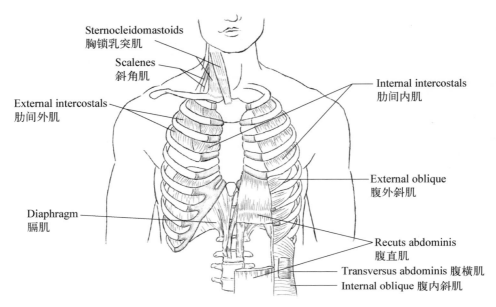

Figure 9–1　The Chest Cavity and Its Contents
（图9–1　胸腔及其内容）

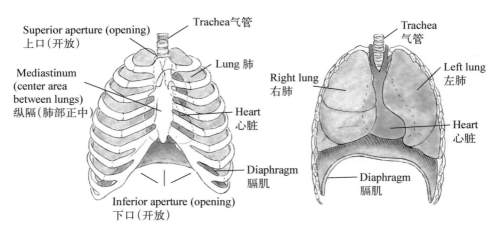

Figure 9–2　The Chest Cavity and Its Contents
（图9–2　胸腔及其内容）

and then pumps it into both lungs through the pulmonary artery for CO_2/O_2 exchange in the lungs. After exchanging, the fresh and oxygenated blood is transported back to the left atrium by the pulmonary vein to complete the pulmonary circulation.

The lungs take up most of the chest space and they connect with the outside through the bronchii, trachea, pharynx and nose to take in oxygen and release carbon dioxide. The basic functional unit in a lung is the alveolus which is an air sac (or like a tiny air bubble). There are about 600 million alveoli in the lungs that would be the size of a tennis court if they were completely stretched out. The surface of each alveolus is covered by surfactant, a chemical compound that is able to maintain the elasticity of the alveoli and the lungs, and consequently prevent the lungs from collapsing. During inspiration, the alveoli puff up to get air in; while during expiration, they shrink to squeeze air out. The segmental (or tertiary) bronchus is the basic anatomical unit of the lung. Each segmental bronchus is separated from the rest of the lung by a connective-tissue septum. Therefore, during pulmonary inflammation, the mucus can be stuck in only one segmental bronchus. Such an anatomical characteristic can be used by a clinician to position a patient properly to perform the cupping technique in order to help the patient discharge the mucus effectively.

The diaphragm is the principle muscle for inspiration. It is a dome-shaped sheet-like muscle with its central part called the central

肺占据了胸腔的大部分空间且通过支气管、气管、咽和鼻子与外部相通，以获取氧气并释放二氧化碳。肺的基本功能单位是肺泡，其是一个囊泡（像一个微小的气泡）。肺里大约有6亿个肺泡，如果将它们完全伸展开，那么它的大小就相当于一个网球场的大小。每个肺泡表面都覆盖着表面活性物质，这是一种能够维持肺泡和肺弹性的化学物质，从而防止肺的塌陷。在吸气时，所有的肺泡都膨胀起来以吸入空气；在呼气时，这些肺泡收缩以排出空气。肺段支气管是肺的基本解剖单位，因为每个肺段都可以通过结缔组织间隔开肺的其他部分。因此，在肺部发炎时，黏液只能滞留在一个肺段内。这样的解剖学特征可以被临床医师用来对患者在适当的体位下进行有效的手法震动治疗，从而有效地排出黏液。

横膈肌是用于呼吸气体的主要肌肉。它是一种穹隆状的肌肉，其中心部位叫作中央肌

tendon and the peripheral part called the muscle belly. When the muscle part contracts, the central tendon is pulled down to increase the chest cavity and make a more negative pressure inside the cavity, which is great for inhaling air into the lungs.

Usually, inspiration is an active process caused by contraction of the diaphragm muscle, while expiration is a passive process caused by the relaxation of the diaphragm due to the elastic recoil ability of the lungs. However, during physical activity time of a healthy person or even during the resting time of a person with medical conditions, the accessary breathing muscles may be needed. There are many accessory inspiratory muscles—such as the external intercostal muscles, the scalene muscles, the sternocleidomastoid muscle, the levator costarum, and the trapezius, in which their contractions can sometimes be observed indicating the utilization of these muscles. There are also accessary expiration muscles like internal intercostal muscles and abdominal muscles. Expiration can be either voluntary or involuntary under different physical conditions. Voluntary expiration is a conscious breathing muscle movement mostly controlled by the motor cortex (e.g., singing a song, or performing a deep breathing exercise at a constant rate). In contrary, involuntary expiration is not a conscious movement and is mainly controlled by the respiratory center located in the pons and medulla (e.g., breathing during sleeping or meditation).

腱,外围部分称为肌腹。当肌肉收缩时,中央肌腱被拉下,胸腔的体积增大,腔内产生更大的负压,有利于肺部吸入空气。

通常,吸气是由膈肌收缩引起的一个主动活动过程,而呼气则是由于肺部的弹性回缩力而导致膈肌自动回位松弛的被动活动过程。然而,在健康人进行身体锻炼时,或者在患者休息时,都可能需要辅助呼吸肌。人体有许多辅助吸气的肌肉,例如肋间外肌、斜角肌、胸锁乳突肌、提肋肌和斜方肌,它们的收缩有时可以被观察到,以表明这些肌肉正被利用。辅助呼气的肌肉有肋间内肌和腹肌。在不同生理条件下,呼气可以是自主的也可以是非自主的。自主呼气是一种有意识的呼吸肌肉运动,主要由运动皮质控制;例如唱歌或者以恒定的速率进行深呼吸训练时。与此相反,非自主的呼气则为无意识的运动,主要由位于脑桥和髓质的呼吸中枢控制,例如在睡觉时或冥想时的呼吸。

New words

thoracic vertebral column　胸椎

sternum ['stɜ:nəm] *n.* 胸骨

diaphragm ['daɪə'fræm] *n.* 膈肌

trachea ['trekɪə] *n.* 气管

esophagus [ɪ'safəgəs] *n.* 食管

chamber ['tʃeɪmbər] *n.* 腔

ventricle ['ventrɪkl] *n.* 心室

atrium ['etrɪəm] *n.* 心房

aorta [e'ɔrtə] *n.* 主动脉

oxygenated blood　含氧血

deoxygenated blood　缺氧血

systematic circulation　体循环

pulmonary ['pʌlmənɛrɪ] *adj.* 肺的

bronchi ['brɑnkaɪ] *n.* 支气管

pharynx ['færɪŋks] *n.* 咽

alveolus [æl'vɪələs] *n.* 肺泡

sac [sæk] *n.* 囊

surfactant [sɜ'fæktənt] *n.* 表面活性剂

elasticity [ˌilæ'stɪsətɪ] *n.* 弹性

collapsing [kə'læpsɪŋ] *adj.* 塌陷的

shrink [ʃrɪŋk] *vt. & vi.* 收缩

squeeze [skwi:z] *vt. & vi.* 挤,挤压

segmental [seg'ment(ə)l] *adj.* 部分的,节段的

connective-tissue septum　结缔组织间隔

mucus ['mjukəs] *n.* 黏液

elastic [ɪ'læstɪk] *adj.* 有弹力的

accessory [ək'sɛsərɪ] *adj.* 附属的

external intercostal muscles　肋间外肌

scalene muscles　斜角肌

sternocleidomastoid muscle　胸锁乳突肌

levator costarum　提肋肌

trapezius [trə'pi:zɪəs] *n.* 斜方肌

utilization [ˌjuːtəlaɪ'zeɪʃn] *n.* 利用, 使用
internal intercostal muscles 肋间内肌
motor cortex 运动皮质
pons and medulla 脑桥和髓质
meditation [ˌmɛdɪ'teʃən] *n.* 冥想

- - - - - - - - - - - - - - - - - - -◀ **Questions** ▶- - - - - - - - - - - - - - - - - - -

❶ Which one of the following structures is not located between the left and right lungs in the chest cavity?

A. The heart.
B. The esophagus.
C. The spleen.
D. The trachea.

❷ The deoxygenated blood is pumped out from _____ into both lungs through the pulmonary artery for CO_2/O_2 exchange in the lungs.

A. the left atrium
B. the left ventricle
C. the right atrium
D. the right ventricle

❸ The basic unit for exchanging oxygen and carbon dioxide in a lung is

_____.

A. the alveolus (plural: alveoli)
B. the primary bronchus (plural: bronchi)
C. the secondary bronchus (Plural: bronchi)
D. the tertiary bronchus (Plural: bronchi)

❹ The diaphragm is the primary muscle for resting inspiration (breathing in). Which one of the following is correct description of this muscle?

A. During inspiration, it moves up toward the chest cavity.
B. During expiration, it moves down toward the abdominal cavity.
C. Its peripheral part is the muscle belly.
D. Its peripheral part is the central tendon.

❺ When you are blowing off 20 birthday candles on your 20-year old birthday, which one of the following muscles do you need to help blow last 2–3 candles off?

A. The serratus anterior muscles (this one should be added to the text).

B. The external intercostal muscle.

C. The abdominal muscles.

D. The sternocleidomastoid muscles.

Answers

❶ C   ❷ D   ❸ A   ❹ C   ❺ C

The Abdominopelvic Cavity
腹盆腔

10

The abdominopelvic cavity (Figure 10-1) is a soda-can like hollow space that contains both the abdominal cavity for the digestive system, kidneys, and adrenal glands, and the pelvic cavity for the urinary system, reproductive system, and the distal part of the digestive tract. Both the superior and inferior boundaries of this cavity are membrane-like, thin and strong muscular structures. The diaphragm, which is dome-like, forms the superior boundary of the abdominopelvic cavity. The pelvic floor (mainly the levator ani muscle), which is shaped like an upside down dome, forms the inferior boundary. Posteromedially, the lumbar and sacral vertebral column is the backbone of the abdominopelvic cavity. The following muscles extend from either side of this column to the anterior abdominal wall: (from posteromedial to anterolateral) psoas major, quadratus lumborum, and abdominal muscles.

The abdominal cavity is much larger than the pelvic cavity. The liver and gallbladder

腹盆腔(图10-1)是一个像易拉罐似的中空的空腔,它容纳了消化系统、肾脏和肾上腺的腹腔以及含泌尿系统、生殖系统和消化道远端的盆腔。腹盆腔的上、下边界均为膜状的薄而有力的肌肉结构:膈肌(穹隆状),形成腹腔的上边界;盆底(主要是肛提肌)呈倒拱状,形成下边界;后中边界是腰椎和骶椎骨性结构,从这脊柱两侧发出而止于腹前臂的肌肉有(从后内侧到前外侧排列)腰大肌、腰方肌和腹肌。

腹腔比盆腔大得多。在腹

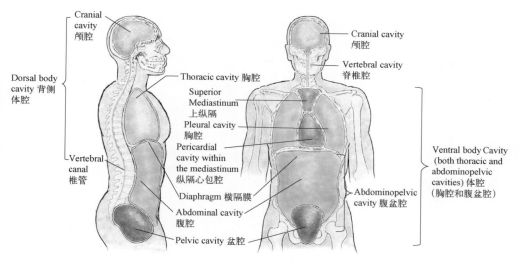

Figure 10–1   The Abdominopelvic cavity

（图10–1   腹盆腔）

are located in the upper right corner of the cavity, and the spleen and stomach are located in the upper left corner. The esophagus passes through the esophageal hiatus of the diaphragm to connect with the stomach, which further connects with the duodenum, jejunum, and ileum. The ileocecal junction, which is located in the lower right corner of the cavity, is where the ileum connects with the ascending colon, then transverse colon, descending colon, sigmoid colon, rectum, and anus at the pelvis. This junction is also where the appendix is located which extends out and downward.

Both left and right kidneys are attached vertically on the posterior wall of the abdominal cavity, with an adrenal gland sitting on top of each kidney. Urine produced by the kidney passes through the ureter to the bladder in the pelvis. When the bladder contracts, the urine

腔内,右上角有肝和胆囊,左上角有脾和胃。食管通过膈上的食管裂孔与胃相连进而与十二指肠、空肠和回肠进一步相连。在右下角处,回盲肠的连接处也是阑尾向下延伸的地方,回肠与升结肠相连,然后升结肠延续为横结肠、降结肠、乙状结肠和盆腔内的直肠和肛门。

左、右肾纵向地贴附于腹腔后壁。肾上腺位于每个肾脏的顶部。肾脏产生的尿液通过输尿管进入盆腔内的膀胱。当膀胱收缩时,膀胱内的尿液最终通过尿道排出。

inside is finally released through the urethra.

The pelvic cavity is a funnel-shaped space that is bounded by pelvic bones. Its pelvic inlet is the superior opening of the pelvis toward the abdomen. The lower boundary of the pelvic cavity is the pelvic floor. In the pelvis, the main organs in males are the bladder, the prostate, the rectum and the anus; and in females, in addition to structures mentioned for the male but excluding the prostate, the cavity also includes the ovaries, the uterine tube, the uterus, and the vagina.

Functionally, we can consider the abdominopelvic cavity as a single hollow air pressure conductor and controller. This conductor is attached to the rigid vertebral column whose stability is supported primarily by the psoas major, the quadratus lumborum, and deep back muscles. On the superior, inferior, lateral, and anterior walls of this conductor are all soft muscles, which are dynamically controlled by the neuromuscular system depending on the body's needs. Enough strength and coordination of these muscles are needed for the abdominopelvic cavity to act as an air pressure controller.

During breathing, particularly during deep breathing, when the diaphragm is pulling down through neuromuscular regulation and coordination, the abdominal muscles, the pelvic floor muscles (levator ani muscle, mainly), and even the back muscles have to be strong enough to ensure stability of other walls of the hollow space, so that the diaphragm can work well on a solid and

盆腔是一个由盆骨构成的漏斗样空间，它的入口是盆骨的上开口通向腹腔；它的下界面是盆底。在骨盆中，男性的主要器官是膀胱、前列腺、直肠和肛门；女性包括的则是除上述男性盆腔中的前列腺外的主要器官以及卵巢、输卵管、子宫和阴道。

在功能上，我们可以把腹盆腔作为一个中空的空气压力导体和控制器。这个导体附着在刚性的椎柱上，它的稳定性主要由腰大肌、腰方肌和背部深层肌肉支撑。在这个导体的上、下面和前壁都是柔软的肌肉，由神经肌肉系统根据身体需要进行动态的控制。腹盆腔作为一个空气压力控制器需要这些肌肉足够的力量强度和相互协调。

在呼吸，特别是深呼吸，膈肌通过神经系统的调控而下降时，腹部肌肉、盆底肌肉（主要是肛提肌），甚至是背部肌肉必须强大到足以确保中空的腹盆腔各壁的稳定，只有这样，膈肌才可以在稳定的稳固的各腹壁支撑下行使功能。否则，如果这些腹壁肌肉都很弱，膈肌就只能在

steady foundation. Otherwise, if other muscles are weak, the diaphragm would have to work on a floppy and unsteady foundation. Consequently, breathing would be affected. In a similar way, during bowel and/or urinary continence, intercourse, or childbirth (in females), the diaphragmatic muscles, pelvic floor muscles, and muscles on the side walls of the abdominopelvic cavity have to be strong enough to maintain a rigid hollow structure for the pelvic muscles to contract solidly. Therefore, for those people with muscle weakness of the diaphragm and/or walls of the abdominopelvic cavity, the pelvic floor muscles may not function well, consequently bowel and/or urinary problems (e.g., retention or incontinence) may occur.

When the balance in strength of these muscles around the abdominopelvic cavity is disturbed or broken, the body may respond with pain or gait abnormality. For example, a gentleman with weak abdominal muscles (e.g., an overweight person) may have lower back pain due to an unbalanced load on his back. He may also experience breathing difficulty and even some dysfunction with bowel and/or urinary activities due to the diaphragm and/or pelvic floor having to work on a floppy foundation.

松软和不稳定的腹壁支撑下工作，进而呼吸就会受到影响。同样，在大小便控制、性生活或分娩（女性）时，盆底肌肉、膈肌以及腹盆腔侧壁上的肌肉也必须足够强大，才能为盆底肌的收缩提供一个稳定的中空刚性结构支撑。所以，对于膈肌和/或腹盆腔侧壁的肌肉力量不足的人来说，他们的盆底肌收缩功能会不好，结果就可能导致大小便的问题（如潴留、失禁）的发生。

当腹盆腔周围肌肉力量平衡被破坏时，身体可能会出现疼痛或步态异常。例如，一个腹部肌肉较弱（如体重超重）的人，由于不平衡的背部过载会导致出现下腰背部痛，也许还会有呼吸困难，甚至大小便活动存在障碍，这都是因为膈肌和/或盆底肌的作用是在一个松软的支撑上的缘故。

New words

abdominopelvic cavity　腹盆腔

soda-can　易拉罐

hollow ['hɒləʊ] *adj.* 中空的

digestive [daɪ'dʒɛstɪv] *adj.* 消化的

adrenal gland　肾上腺

pelvic cavity ['pelvɪk'kæviti] *n.* 盆腔

urinary ['jʊərɪnərɪ] *adj.* 泌尿的

reproductive system　生殖系统

pelvic floor ['pelvɪkflɔː] *n.* 盆底

levator ani muscle　肛提肌

posteromedial [ˌpɒstərə'medɪəl] *adj.* 后内侧的

anterolateral [æntərəʊ'leɪtərəl] *adj.* 前外侧的

psoas major　腰大肌

quadratus lumborum　腰方肌

gall bladder [gɔːl'blædə] *n.* 胆囊

spleen [spliːn] *n.* 脾

esophageal hiatus [ˌiːsə'fædʒɪəhaɪ'eɪtəs] *n.* 食管裂孔

duodenum ['dʊə'dɪnəm] *n.* 十二指肠

jejunum [dʒɪ'dʒunəm] *n.* 空肠

ileum ['ɪlɪəm] *n.* 回肠

ileocecal junction　回盲结合部

ascending colon *n.* 升结肠

transverse colon *n.* 横结肠

descending colon *n.* 降结肠

sigmoid colon *n.* 乙状结肠

rectum ['rɛktəm] *n.* 直肠

anus ['enəs] *n.* 肛门

appendix [ə'pɛndɪks] *n.* 阑尾

ureter [jʊ'riːtə] *n.* 输尿管

bladder ['blædə(r)] *n.* 膀胱

urethra [jʊ'riːθrə] *n.* 尿道

prostate ['prɑstet] *n.* 前列腺

ovaries [ovərɪz] *n.* 卵巢（复数）

uterine tube ['juːtəraintjuːb] *n.* 输卵管

uterus ['jutərəs] *n.* 子宫

vagina [vəˈdʒaɪnə] *n.* 阴道

floppy [ˈflɑpɪ] *adj.* 松软的

intercourse [ˈɪntəkɔrs] *n.* 性交

retention [rɪˈtenʃn] *n.* 潴留

incontinence [ɪnˈkɒntɪnəns] *n.* 失禁

---------------------------◀ **Questions** ▶----------------------------

❶ On the abdominal wall, which one of the following muscles is most posteriorly and medially located?

A. The psoas major muscle.

B. The quadratus lumborum muscle.

C. The abdominal muscles.

D. The levator ani muscle.

❷ Which one of the following structures is located in the upper right corner of the abdominal cavity?

A. The stomach.　　　　　　　　　B. The spleen.

C. The gall bladder.　　　　　　　　D. The appendix.

❸ Which one of the following structures exists only in the male but not in the female human body?

A. The bladder.　　　　　　　　　　B. The rectum.

C. The prostate.　　　　　　　　　　D. The anus.

❹ The adrenal gland is located on top of _____.

A. the spleen　　　　　　　　　　　B. the liver

C. the pancreas　　　　　　　　　　D. the kidney

❺ The abdominopelvic cavity is like an air pressure cylinder. When one is trying very hard to breathing out as much as possible, what do you expect his pelvic floor muscle to do to help the expiration?

A. The pelvic floor muscle contracts and moves down to increase the abdominopelvic pressure in order for the diaphragm to move up.

B. The pelvic floor muscle contracts and moves up to increase the abdominopelvic pressure in order for the diaphragm to move up.

C. The pelvic floor muscle relaxes and moves down to increase the abdominopelvic pressure in order for the diaphragm to move up.

D. The pelvic floor muscle contracts and moves up to decrease the abdominopelvic pressure in order for the diaphragm to move up.

Answers

❶ A   ❷ C   ❸ C   ❹ D   ❺ B

The Upper Extremity
上肢

11

As human beings evolved from the quadruped posture to the bipedal one, their upper and lower extremities develop gradually and differently in functionality. A person's upper extremity (UE) progresses to be responsible for manipulative activities, while the lower extremity (LE) progresses to be for body weight support and ambulation. In other words, the UE primarily performs open-chain activities in which the proximal portion of a limb is stable while the distal portion is mobile. In contrary, the LE performs closed-chain activities, in which the proximal portion of the limb is mobile, while the distal portion is stable.

The UE (Figure 11–1 and Figure 11–2) includes the upper arm, the forearm, and the hand. As the proximal portion of the UE, the upper arm is connected to the trunk through the shoulder girdle and shoulder joint. The shoulder girdle includes the clavicle and the scapula. The shoulder joint (also known as the glenohumeral joint or GH joint) is a

在人类由四足动物进化成为两足动物的进化过程中，上肢和下肢逐渐在功能方面产生了差异。人体的上肢逐渐发展为主要负责精细活动，而下肢负责承重和步行。换言之，上肢主要进行近端固定远端活动的开链运动；相反，下肢则进行近端活动远端固定的闭链运动。

上肢（图11-1和图11-2）包括上臂、前臂和手。作为上肢的近端部分，上臂通过肩带和肩关节与躯干相连接。肩带包括锁骨和肩胛骨。肩关节（也被称为盂肱关节或GH关节）是由肱骨上呈凸面的肱骨头和肩胛骨上呈凹面的关节盂组成的滑膜球

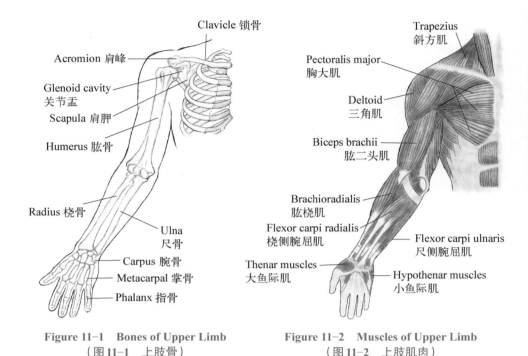

Figure 11-1　Bones of Upper Limb
（图 11-1　上肢骨）

Figure 11-2　Muscles of Upper Limb
（图 11-2　上肢肌肉）

synovial ball-and-socket joint formed between the big convex head of the humerus and the concave glenoid cavity of the scapula. Scapular movement on the posterior rib cage is required to raise the arms overhead. The GH joint is stabilized by many ligaments and muscles anteriorly, superiorly, and posteriorly around the joint. The rotator cuff muscles, including the supraspinatus, infraspinatus, teres minor, and subscapularis, is a group of muscles to stabilize the GH joint. This joint acts like a lever to move the entire UE in different directions in a 3-D space. During the UE movement, the shoulder joint must be stable to ensure accurate execution of tasks by distal joints. For example, when someone is

窝关节。当手臂抬高过头顶时，需要肩胛骨在胸廓后壁上的运动相配合。盂肱关节被关节周围前方、上方和后方的肌肉和韧带加固。包括冈上肌、冈下肌、小圆肌和肩胛下肌的肩袖肌群是一组稳定盂肱关节的肌肉。上肢运动时，肩关节如同杠杆一样确保整个上肢在三维空间里不同方向上的运动。例如，当投篮时，上肢面向前方，肩关节必须保持稳定才能确保手恰当地执行投篮动作。

shooting a basketball, the UE faces anteriorly, and the shoulder joint has to be stable to ensure the proper hand execution of ball-shooting.

The middle portion of the UE includes the elbow joint that is comprised of three joints within one synovial capsule: the humeroradial, the humeroulnar, and the proximal radioulnar joints. Together with the distal radioulnar joint, these four joints act together to place the hand in a desirable position to perform various tasks. The action of these joints is made possible by the muscles around them. For instance, when you hold a basketball on the left hand and push the ball out with your right hand to shoot the ball, your right shoulder, elbow and forearm will have to be steadily positioned in order for the hand to execute the shooting action accurately.

The distal portion of the UE includes the wrist, the carpometacarpal joints, the metacarpophalangeal joints, and the interphalangeal joints. These joints work together to ensure the final accuracy of the hand and fingers on target or for performing the task dexterously. In the same example of shooting a basketball, the hand and fingers will be the final components to execute the shooting accuracy. In terms of dexterity, the index and middle fingers are mostly used for precision work like writing and painting. The ring and little fingers are mostly used for grip work like holding a cup.

As you can see from above, along the chain of the UE joints, mobility and stability

上肢中间部分的肘关节包括包裹在1个关节囊内的3个关节：肱桡关节、肱尺关节和桡尺近侧关节。加上桡尺远侧关节，这4个关节共同作用，使手处于完成不同任务时所需要的摆放位置，这些关节的运动是通过其周围的肌肉来实现的。例如，当你用左手握住篮球并用右手将球推射投球时，你的右肩、肘和前臂必须稳定定位，以确保手能准确地执行投篮动作。

上肢远端包括腕关节、腕掌关节、掌指关节和指间关节。这些关节一起工作以保证手和手指完成特定动作时最后所需的精准性或手指灵敏性。依然以投篮为例，手和手指是投篮动作精确执行的最后部分。在手指灵敏性方面，示指和中指用于完成精细运动如写字和绘画；而无名指和小手指则用于抓握活动如紧握住1个杯子。

正如上文所述，在上肢的关节链上，上肢近端部分（如肩关

of the proximal portions of the UE (e.g., the shoulder and elbow joint) are the prerequisites for the distal portion of the UE (e.g., the hand and fingers) to be desirably placed in order to execute actions accurately and functionally.

The big muscles of the UE are close to the trunk and provide stability and mobility. Around the shoulder and arm, there are the pectoralis major on the front and latissimus dorsi on the back; and the biceps brachii in the anterior and the triceps brachii in the posterior compartments of the arm. Muscles in the forearm and hand are smaller and more slender, including the flexor digitorum superficialis and profundus and extensor digitorum on the forearm; and many intrinsic muscles in the hand used for detailed dexterity.

节、肘关节)的灵活性和稳定性是让远端部分(手和手指)置于合适位置并准确完成所需动作和功能执行的先决条件。

上肢的大肌肉靠近躯干并提供稳定性和活动度。在肩关节和手臂周围,有主要位于前面的胸大肌和背部的背阔肌,手臂前部的肱二头肌和后部的肱三头肌。前臂和手部的肌肉,更小更纤细,包括位于前臂负责灵活性的指浅屈肌、指深屈肌、指伸肌和很多在手上用于精细活动的手固有肌。

New words

evolve v. 进化,进展
quadruped ['kwɑdrupɛd] adj. 有四足的,四脚的,四点的
posture ['pɑstʃɚ] n. 姿势
bipedal [baɪ'pɛdəl] adj. 两足的,二足的,二点的
extremities [iks'tremɪtɪs] n. 肢体,极限(extremity复数形式)
upper and lower extremities　上下肢
manipulative [mə'nɪpjəletɪv] adj. 巧妙处理的,操纵的,用手控制的
ambulation [ˌæmbju-'leɪʃən] n. 移动,步行
open-chain　开链
proximal ['prɑksɪməl] adj. 近端的,近身体中央的
portion ['pɔrʃən] n. 部分
proximal portion　近端部分
limb [lɪm] n. 肢,臂
distal ['dɪstl] adj. 末端的,远端的

distal portion　远端部分

mobile ['məʊbl]　*adj.* 可移动的，机动的

upper arm　上臂

forearm ['fɔːrɑːm]　*n.* 前臂

trunk [trʌŋk]　*n.* 树干，躯干

shoulder girdle　肩胛带

clavicle ['klævəkl]　*n.* 锁骨

scapula ['skæpjələ]　*n.* 肩胛，肩胛骨

glenohumeral (GH) joint　盂肱关节

synovial [sɪ'nəʊviəl]　*adj.* 滑液的，分泌滑液的

socket ['sɑkɪt]　*n.* 插座；窝，穴；牙槽

ball-and-socket joint　球窝关节

convex ['kɑnvɛks]　*adj.* 凸的，凸面的

humerus ['hjumərəs]　*n.* 肱骨

concave [kɑn'kev]　*adj.* 凹的，凹面的

glenoid ['gliːnɔɪd]　*adj.* 浅窝的；关节窝的

cavity ['kævəti]　*n.* 腔；洞，凹处

glenoid cavity　关节盂

posteriorly [pɒs'tɪɔriəlɪ]　*adv.* 后来的，其次的，后面的

rib [rɪb]　*n.* 肋骨

posterior rib cage　后胸腔

ligament ['lɪgəmənt]　*n.* 韧带

anteriorly [æn'tɪriːəlɪ]　*adv.* 先前的，前面的，在前面

superiorly [sjuː'pɪərɪəlɪ]　*adv.* 上面的，在上面

rotator ['rotetɚ]　*n.* 旋转体，旋转的人回旋肌

rotator cuff　肩袖

supraspinatus　*n.* 冈上肌，棘上肌

infraspinatus　冈下肌

teres ['te.riːz]　*n.* 圆肌

teres minor　小圆肌

subscapularis ['sʌb'skæpju'lɛərɪs]　*n.* 肩胛下肌

lever ['lɛvɚ]　*n.* 杠杆；控制杆　*vt.* 用杠杆撬动；把……作为杠杆

execute ['ɛksɪkjut]　*vt.* 实行；执行；处死

execution [ˌɛksɪ'kjuʃən] *n.* 执行，实行；完成

ensure accurate execution 确保准确执行

capsule ['kæpsl;] *n.* 胶囊

synovial capsule 滑膜囊

humeroradial *adj.* 肱桡的

humeroulnar 肱尺的

radioulnar [ˌreɪdɪəu'ʌlnə] *adj.* 桡尺骨的

desirable [dɪ'zaɪərəbl] *adj.* 令人满意的；值得要的 *n.* 合意的人或事

carpometacarpal *adj.* 腕掌的，腕骨与掌间的

metacarpophalangeal *adj.* 掌指的

interphalangeal joint 指间关节，趾间关节

dexterously ['dɛkstrɔrslɪ] *adv.* 巧妙地；敏捷地

dexterity [dɛk'stɛrətɪ] *n.* 灵巧；敏捷；机敏

component [kəm'ponənt] *n.* 成分；组件

In terms of 依据；按照

index and middle fingers 示指和中指

precision [prɪ'sɪʒn] *n.* 精度，*adj.* 精密的，精确的

the ring and little fingers 环指和小指

prerequisite [ˌprɪ'rɛkwəzɪt] *n.* 先决条件；*adj.* 首要必备的

pectoralis ['pektərəlɪs] *n.* 胸肌

latissimus dorsi 背阔肌

biceps ['baɪsɛps] *n.* 二头肌

brachii （拉）臂

biceps brachii 肱二头肌

triceps brachii 肱三头肌

slender ['slɛndə] *adj.* 细长的；苗条的；微薄的

digitorum 趾的

profundus [pro'fʌndəs] *n.* 深屈肌

❮ Questions ❯

❶ Which one of the following activities is considered as the close-chain activity of the upper extremity?

A. To pick up a trash can from the floor.

B. To grab a tea cup on the table.

C. To perform a push-up on the floor.

D. To receive a parcel from a delivery person.

❷ The rotator cuff muscles are a group of muscles that are able to stabilize

_____.

A. the scapular movement on the rib cage

B. the humeral head on the glenoid cavity of the scapula

C. the sternum on the clavicle

D. the clavicle on the acromion of the scapula

❸ Which one of the following joint groups is within the same joint capsule?

A. The humeroradial joint, the humeroulnar joint, and the proximal radioulnar joint.

B. The humeroradial joint, the humeroulnar joint, and the distal radioulnar joint.

C. The humeroradial joint, the proximal and distal radioulnar joints.

D. The humeroulnar joint, the proximal and distal radioulnar joints.

❹ When you are shooting a basketball to the hoop, which one of the joint's stability is critical for the whole upper limb to perform the shooting action accurately?

A. The finger joints.   B. The wrist joint.

C. The elbow joint.   D. The shoulder joint.

❺ Which one of the following actions is considered not to be the main action of the index and middle fingers?

A. Using a pair of chopsticks.

B. Writing a sentence with a pencil.

C. Painting a picture in detail.

D. Griping a water cup tightly.

Answers ·········

❶ C   ❷ B   ❸ A   ❹ D   ❺ D

The Lower Extremity
下肢

12

The lower extremity (LE) includes the thigh, the leg, and the foot, which are connected by the hip, knee, and ankle joints (Figure 12–1 and Figure 12–2). The main function of the LE is to support body weight and maintain proper body posture during standing and walking.

The thigh is attached to the pelvic bone through the hip joint which is a synovial ball-and-socket joint between the femoral head and the acetabulum of the hipbone. Similar to the shoulder joint, the hip joint allows a large degree of multidirectional movements in a 3-D space. There are ligaments and muscles around the joint that act to maintain stability and mobility. Among the muscles, the gluteus medius and minimus may act, somehow like the "rotator cuff" muscles for the shoulder joint, to stabilize as well as to move the hip joint. Both the gluteus medius with its anterior, middle, and posterior parts and the gluteus minimus with its two parts cover and stabilize the hip joint by inserting on the greater trochanter of the femur.

下肢(LE)包括大腿、小腿和足部,通过髋关节、膝关节和踝关节相连接(图12-1和图12-2),其主要功能是支撑身体的重量,在站立和行走时保持适当的身体姿势。

大腿与骨盆骨通过髋关节相连,髋关节是股骨头和髋骨髋臼之间的滑膜球窝关节。与肩关节类似,髋关节在三维空间中允许有很大程度的多方向运动。关节周围有韧带和肌肉以保持其稳定性和移动性。在肌肉中,臀中肌和臀小肌的作用有点像"肩关节肩袖"肌肉,以稳定和活动髋关节。臀中肌的前、中、后部分和臀小肌的两部分止于股骨的大转子,覆盖及稳定髋关节。

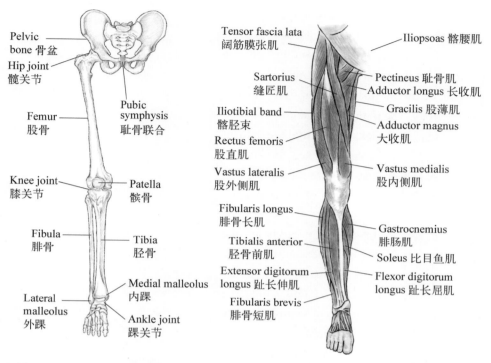

Figure 12–1   Bones of Lower limb
（图12–1   下肢骨）

Figure 12–2   Muscles of Lower limb
（图12–2   下肢肌肉）

Moving down to the knee, the femur articulates with the tibia and the patella to make the tibiofemoral and the patellofemoral joints. The tibiofemoral joint is the main part of the knee joint that is stabilized by the medial and lateral collateral ligaments (MCL and LCL) outside the joint capsule and the anterior and posterior cruciate ligaments (ACL and PCL) inside the joint. On the tibial surface of the knee joint are the medial and lateral menisci that function to disperse the body weight and minimize friction between the two joint surfaces when the joint is holding a load like during standing or walking. The

　　下到膝关节，股骨与胫骨和髌骨连接，构成胫股关节和髌股关节。胫股关节是膝关节的主要部分，由关节囊外的内、外侧副韧带（MCL和LCL）和关节内前、后交叉韧带（ACL和PCL）提供稳定性。关节的胫骨表面是内侧和外侧半月板，当关节承受负荷时，比如站立和行走时，其作用是分散身体的重量，并尽量减少两个关节面之间的摩擦。髌骨位于股骨髁间沟内，形成髌股关节，其具有稳定髌骨腱，减轻关节表面的压力，提高股四头

patella lies within the intercondylar groove of the femur to form the patellofemoral joint which stabilizes the patellar tendon, reduces pressure on the joint surfaces, and increases the power of the quadriceps muscle during knee activity. The main movement of the knee is to extend and flex, and can also perform medial and lateral rotation when the knee is flexed. A healthy patellofemoral joint is the indispensable prerequisite of normal knee movement.

Between the knee and the ankle are the larger tibia medially and the smaller fibula laterally. These two bones are connected by two slightly movable articulations: the proximal tibiofibular one−a synovial plane joint; and the distal tibiofibular one−a non-synovial syndesmosis joint. Further down, the distal surface of both the tibia and fibula form a mortise-like concave surface to articulate with the convex superior surface of the talus forming the ankle joint. The architectural arrangement permits dorsiflexion and plantar flexion of the ankle joint in the sagittal plane.

Immediately below the ankle joint is the subtalar joint between the talus and the calcaneus, which is the most inferior joint of the LE where both bones are in the vertical plane. From here forward joints in the horizontal plane include the midtarsal joints (among the tarsal bones), the tarsometatarsal joints, the metatarsophalangeal joints, and the interphalangeal joints. All the joints from the ankle down to the toes, which are united

肌在膝关节活动中的爆发力的作用。膝关节的主要运动是伸和屈,当屈曲位时膝关节还可以进行内旋和外旋。健康的髌股关节是膝关节正常运动不可或缺的前提。

在膝关节和踝关节之间是位于内侧大的胫骨和外侧小的腓骨。这2块骨头是由2个可略微移动性的关节相连:近端胫腓骨连接是一个滑膜平面关节;以及远端胫腓骨连接是一个非滑膜的联合关节。进一步向下,胫骨和腓骨的远端表面形成一种类似于榫眼的凹表面,与距骨上凸面相连形成的踝关节。这种结构可以使踝关节在矢状面背屈和跖屈。

踝关节下面的是距骨和跟骨之间的距下关节,它是下肢在垂直平面上的最下端关节。从这里向前在水平平面内的关节包括中跗骨间关节(在跗骨中)、跗跖关节、跖趾关节和趾间关节。从踝关节到脚趾的所有关节由许多致密的韧带紧紧连接,使脚能够在三维空间内恰当且协调地活动,这种肌动学特性保

by many tight ligaments, work coordinately and properly to enable the foot to move in 3-D planes. This kinematical characteristic of the foot ensures that each individual part of the foot adjusts for different weight-bearing situations. For example, one has to adjust the weight-bearing foot to response to the ground reaction force (during the stance phase) when walking on an uneven pebble trail, tiptoe jumping, or single-leg standing on a beam.

There are many muscles in the LE, including the quadriceps in the front of the thigh; the hamstrings in the back of the thigh; the tibialis anterior, the extensor digitorum, and the extensor halluces in the front of the lower leg; and the calf muscles, tibialis posterior, the flexor digitorum, and the flexor halluces in the back of the lower leg. Actions of the LE muscles provide foundational stability for upright posture during standing. They also coordinate the chain reaction of the LE joints by creating appropriate power, range of motion, and velocity of muscle contractions for correct gait pattern during ambulation.

证了脚的每一部分都能为不同身体负重的情形进行调整。例如，当行走在不平坦的鹅卵石小道上，或踮起脚尖跳跃，或单腿站立在横梁上时，一个人必须调整（支撑相）承重脚的反应以适应地面的反作用力。

下肢有很多肌肉，包括大腿前部的股四头肌，大腿后面的腘绳肌，小腿前面的胫骨前肌、趾伸肌以及踇趾伸肌，还有小腿后面的腓肠肌、胫骨后肌、趾屈肌和踇趾屈肌。在站立时，下肢肌肉的活动为直立姿势提供了功能稳定性。它们还通过产生适度的力量、活动范围和肌肉收缩的速度来协调下肢步行过程中的运动链反应以达到正确的步态模式。

New words

thigh [θaɪ] *n.* 大腿,股
pelvic ['pɛlvɪk] *adj.* 骨盆的
synovial [sɪ'nəuvɪəl] *adj.* 滑液的
socket ['sakɪt] *n.* 窝,穴；牙槽
ball-and-socket joint　球窝关节
femoral ['femərəl] *adj.* 股骨的；大腿的

acetabulum [ˌæsə'tæbjʊləm] *n.* 髋臼；关节窝

hipbone ['hɪpˌbon] *n.* 臀骨；髋骨

multidirectional [ˌmʌltɪdaɪ'rɛkʃənəl] *adj.* 多方向的

3-Dimensional [daɪ'mɛnʃənl] 三维空间的

gluteus ['glutɪəs] *n.* 臀肌

medius ['miːdɪəs] *n.* 中指；中间的东西

minimus ['mɪnɪməs] *n.* 最小的东西

gluteus medius and minimus　臀中肌和臀小肌

rotator cuff　肩袖

insert *v.* 插入，嵌进，肌肉止于……

trochanter [tro'kæntɚ] *n.* 转子；粗隆

greater trochanter of the femur　股骨大转子

articulate [ɑr'tɪkjulet] *vt.* 用关节连接；使相互连贯

tibia ['tɪbɪə] *n.* 胫骨

patella [pə'tɛlə] 髌骨

tibiofemoral [ˌtibiəu'femərəl] *adj.* 胫股的

patellofemoral [pəˌtelə'femərəl] *adj.* 髌股的

collateral [kə'lætərəl] *adj.* 旁系的；附属的

medial and lateral collateral ligaments（MCL 和 LCL）　内侧和外侧副韧带

cruciate ['kruːʃɪət; -eɪt] *adj.* 十字状的，十字形的

anterior and posterior cruciate ligaments（ACL 和 PCL）　前、后交叉韧带

menisci [mɪ'nɪsaiˌ-kai] *n.* 半月板；新月形物（meniscus 的复数形式）

intercondylar　髁间的；踝间的

groove [gruv] *n.* 凹槽

tendon ['tɛndən] *n.* 腱

quadriceps ['kwɑdrəsɛps] *n.* 股四头肌

rotation [ro'teʃən] *n.* 旋转；循环，轮流

medial and lateral rotation　内外侧旋转

fibula ['fɪbjələ] *n.* 腓骨

syndesmosis [ˌsɪndɛs'mosɪs] *n.* 韧带联合

mortise ['mɔrtɪs] *n.* 榫眼

concave [kɑn'kev] *n.* 凹面；*adj.* 凹的，凹面的

convex ['kɑnvɛks] *n.* 凸面体；凸状；*adj.* 凸面的

talus ['teɪləs] *n.* 距骨；踝；斜面

architectural [ˌɑrkɪ'tɛktʃərəl] *adj.* 建筑上的，结构上的

dorsiflexion [ˌdɔːsɪ'flekʃən] *n.* 背屈

plantar ['plæntə] *adj.* 跖的

plantar flexion 跖屈

sagittal ['sædʒətl] *adj.* 矢状的

sagittal plane 矢状平面

subtalar 距下的

calcaneus [kæl'kenɪəs] *n.* 跟骨

vertical plane 垂直面

horizontal plane 水平平面

tarsal ['tɑːsəl] *n.* 跗骨；*adj.* 跗骨的

tarsometatarsal joints 跗跖关节

metatarsophalangeal 跖趾的

metatarsophalangeal joints 跖趾关节

interphalangeal *adj.* 指节间的

interphalangeal joints 趾间关节，指间关节

kinematical *adj.* 运动学的

stance phase 承重相，支撑相

uneven pebble trail 凹凸不平的鹅卵石小道

tiptoe ['tɪpto] *n.* 脚尖；趾尖

beam [bim] *n.* 横梁，平衡木

hamstring ['hæmstrɪŋ] 腘绳肌

tibialis anterior 胫骨前肌

extensor [ɪk'stɛnsə] *n.* 伸肌

digitorum 趾的

extensor digitorum 指伸肌

halluces ['hæljusiːz] *n.* 大拇趾；后趾（hallux 的复数）

extensor halluces 伸肌后趾

calf [kæf] *n.* 腓肠，小腿

calf muscles 腓肠肌群

tibialis posterior 胫骨后肌

flexor ['flɛksə] *n.* 屈肌

flexor digitorum　趾屈肌
flexor halluces　踇趾屈肌
upright ['ʌpraɪt]　*n.* 垂直；直立；*adj.* 垂直的，直立的
upright posture　直立姿势
velocity [və'lɑsətɪ]　*n.* 速度
contraction [kən'trækʃən]　*n.* 收缩，紧缩
pattern ['pætərn]　*n.* 模式；图案
gait pattern　步态模式
ambulation [ˌæmbju-'leɪʃən]　*n.* 移动；步行

--------------------------- **Questions** ---------------------------

1 Which one of the following muscles is having its muscle fibers surrounding the hip joint anteriorly, laterally, and posteriorly and be able to stabilize the joint?

A. The gluteus maximus. 　　　　B. The gluteus medius.

C. The gluteus minimus. 　　　　D. The tensor fascia lata.

2 Speaking of the ACL, the letter "C" stands for "_____".

A. Central 　　　　B. Continous

C. Cruciate 　　　　D. Collateral

3 The mortise-like concave surface for the ankle joint is very important for stabilizing the joint. This surface is usually formed by _____.

A. the tibia 　　　　B. the fibula

C. the talus 　　　　D. both the fibula and tibia

4 On the vertical plane, which one of the following choices is the lowest one?

A. The ankle joint. 　　　　B. The subtalar joint.

C. The metatarsophalangeal joint. 　　　　D. The interphalangeal joint.

❺ The name for the group of muscles in the back of the thigh is _____ .

    A. the quadriceps   B. the tibialis

    C. the calf   D. the hamstrings

Answers

❶ B   ❷ C   ❸ D   ❹ B   ❺ D

Basics and Application of Body Mechanics

人体力学的基础和应用

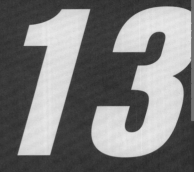

The skeleton is the only system that is able to provide a rigid frame to hold and protect other systems, to support body weight, and to move the body via its joints. In body mechanics, a bone is like a lever in physics that is able to move around a joint (called a fulcrum in physics). The rigid bone frame is covered by muscles that allow movement by pulling on bones. The type, extent, and efficiency of a bone movement can be determined by the load or resistance applied to the bone (the lever).

The following are the 3 classes of levers in the human body:

1. A first class lever (Figure 13–1) is when the fulcrum (axis) lies between the muscle pulling effort/force and the load/resistance. A good example is the atlanto-occipital joint as the fulcrum where the weight of the head is the load (resistance) and the muscles at the back of the head are the effort force (which prevents the head from bending down anteriorly). This type of lever is seen the least in the body.

骨骼是能够提供刚性框架来支撑和保护身体其他系统，支撑身体重量，并能通过关节来移动身体的唯一系统。在人体力学中，骨头的作用就像物理学中的杠杆，能够绕着一个关节（物理学中称为支点）来运动。刚性的骨骼框架通过覆盖其上的肌肉拉动骨头产生运动。骨运动的类型、程度和效率可由施加于骨（杠杆）的负荷或阻力来决定。

下面介绍的是人体中的三类杠杆：

1. 第一类杠杆（图13–1），是当支点（轴）位于肌肉拉力/动力作用点和负载/阻力作用点之间。一个很好的例子是寰枕关节作为支点，头部的重量是负荷，头部后方的肌肉是动力（防止头部向前下弯曲），这种类型的杠杆在身体中是最少的。

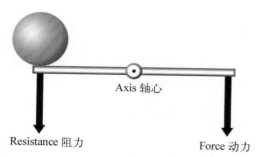

Axis 轴心

Resistance 阻力   Force 动力

Figure 13–1   **A first class lever–the fulcrum (axis) lies between the muscle pulling effort/force and the load/resistance**

（图 13-1   第一类杠杆：支点、轴位于肌肉拉力／动力和负荷／阻力之间）

2. A second class lever (Figure 13–2) is when the resistance is between the fulcrum and the muscle force. For example, when tiptoe standing, the point where the toes contact the ground is the fulcrum, the body weight is the load/resistance at the ankle joint area (to lower the heel down), and the calf muscles for plantar flexion are the muscle effort force (to prevent the heel from lowering down).

2. 第二类杠杆（图 13-2），是阻力作用点位于支点和肌肉动力作用点之间。例如，当踮起脚尖站立时，脚趾接触地面的点是支点，负荷／阻力是作用于踝关节区域的身体重量（拉脚跟向下），而用于跖屈的小腿肌肉提供动力（防止脚跟向下）。

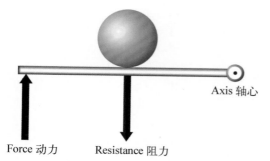

Axis 轴心

Force 动力   Resistance 阻力

Figure 13–2   **A second class lever–the load is located between the fulcrum and the muscle effort**

（图 13-2   第二类杠杆：负荷位于支点和肌肉动力之间）

3. A third class lever (Figure 13–3), the most common one in the human body, is when the muscle force lies between the resistance (load) and the fulcrum. For instance, when performing a biceps curl with a dumbbell, the elbow is the fulcrum, the dumbbell is the resistance, and the biceps brachii muscle makes the effort to bend the forearm.

3. 第三类杠杆（图13–3），人体中最常见的一种，是当肌肉动力作用点位于阻力（负荷）作用点和支点之间时。举个例子，当手持哑铃收缩肱二头肌屈曲肘关节时，肘关节是支点，哑铃是阻力，肱二头肌提供前臂弯曲的肌肉动力。

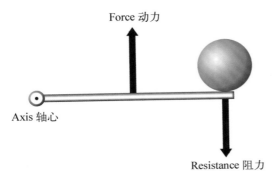

Force 动力

Axis 轴心

Resistance 阻力

Figure 13–3　A third class lever–the muscle effort lies between the resistance (load) and the fulcrum

（图13–3　第三类杠杆：肌肉的动力处于阻力/负荷之间）

When performing any body movement, one needs to use proper body mechanics (Figure 13–4) to minimize stress and strain injuries on the body. When moving a heavy object, a person should use muscles near the body to complete the task. For example, using shoulders, upper arms, hips and/or thighs to move the object, rather than the forearms, hands, legs and/or toes. Use of these near-the-trunk muscles allows the body's center of gravity (COG) to fall within the base of support (BOS), which is usually the area between the two feet. If at any time when

在身体运动时，很有必要利用适当的人体力学特征来减轻身体的应力性与牵拉性损伤（图13–4）。当搬运重物时，人体应该用靠近身体的肌肉来完成工作。例如，使用肩关节、上臂、髋关节和/或大腿来移动物体，而不是前臂、手、腿和/或脚趾。使用这些接近躯干的肌肉可以让身体的重心（COG）落于位于两脚之间的区域，即支撑面（BOS）内。任何时间在搬起重物时，如果重心超出支撑面的范围，就可

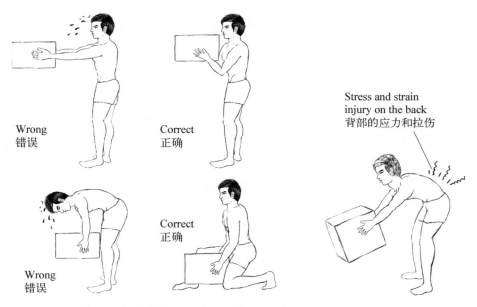

Stress and strain
injury on the back
背部的应力和拉伤

Wrong
错误

Correct
正确

Correct
正确

Wrong
错误

Figure 13-4   The posture of lifting a heavy box from the floor
（图13-4   从地面搬运重物的姿势）

lifting a heavy load, the COG is out of the boundary of the BOS, an injury may occur to the person's back.

On a daily basis, we do a lot of lifting, moving, and carrying items. During these activities, proper body mechanics should always be emphasized, particularly for those who perform strenuous jobs. Let's look at an example here. When someone tries to lift a heavy box from the floor, he or she is actually practicing a first class lever activity. The fulcrum is the vertebral column, which sits on the pelvis with the lumbosacral junction (LSJ) between the L5 and the S1 vertebrae. The resistance (R) is the heavy box. The lever length for the resistance (L_R) is the distance from the box to the LSJ. While on the other hand, the effort force (E) is

能会导致搬物者的背部受伤。

在日常生活中，我们会做大量的抬举、移动和搬运物品的动作。在这些活动中，应该始终强调适当的人体力学，尤其是那些从事艰苦体力工作的人。让我们看一个例子，当有人试图从地板上举起一个沉重的箱子时，他或她实际上是在练习第一种类型的杠杆活动。支点位于脊柱上L5与S1之间的腰骶关节连接处。阻力（R）是重箱子。阻力臂（LR）是从箱子重力作用线到腰骶交界处的垂直距离。而在另一方面，动力（E）由竖脊肌提供，而动力臂（LE）是从肌

the erector spinae muscle, and the lever length of the effort force (L_E) is the very short distance from the muscle to the LSJ. By looking at the formula with two torques equalized ($T_R = T_E$), namely, $R \times L_R = E \times L_E$, we can see that the longer the L_R is, the more strength required from the muscle effort, since the L_E is unchangeable. Therefore, it is understandable that when we lift something heavy, we need to bend the knees, keep the back straight, spread the feet at least one foot apart, use leg muscles, and hold the object close to the body to shorten the L_R length. If a turning action is needed, one should turn the whole body instead of twisting the trunk. By performing all of these, we can avoid unnecessary stress or strain injury and minimize potential harm to our backs.

肉拉力作用线到腰骶交界处的非常短的距离。通过观察这个两力矩平衡公式（$T_R=T_E$），即 $R \times L_R=E \times L_E$，我们可以看出阻力臂越长，所需的肌力越大，因为 L_E（肌肉动力臂）长度是不可改变的。因此，可以理解的是，当我们抬起重物时，我们需要弯曲膝盖，保持背部挺直，双脚分开至少一脚的距离，使用腿部肌肉，将物体紧贴身体以缩短阻力臂（L_R）长度。如果需要转体动作，请转动整个身体，而不是扭动躯干。通过所有这些，我们可以避免背部不必要的应力或牵拉性损伤以及减少潜在的伤害风险。

New words

skeleton ['skɛlɪtn] *n.* 骨架

rigid ['rɪdʒɪd] *adj.* 严格的；刚性的，坚硬的

rigid frame　刚性构架

via ['viːə] *prep.* 通过；经由

fulcrum ['fʊlkrəm] *n.* 支点

lever ['lɛvə] *n.* 杠杆；控制杆

axis ['æksɪs/] *n.* 轴；轴线

load [lod] *n.* 负载，负荷；*vt.* 使担负；装填

resistance [rɪ'zɪstəns] *n.* 阻力

atlanto-occipital　寰枕的

tiptoe ['tɪpto] *n.* 脚尖

calf muscles　腓肠肌群

plantar ['plæntə] *adj.* 跖的

plantar flexion　跖屈

bicep curl　屈臂

dumbbell ['dʌmbel] *n.* 哑铃

biceps brachii muscle　肱二头肌

body mechanics　人体力学

strain [stren] *n.* 张力，牵张，肌肉拉伤

strenuous ['strɛnjuəs] *adj.* 紧张的；费力的

vertebrae ['vɜ:tɪbreɪ] *n.* 椎骨；脊椎

vertebral column　脊柱

pelvis ['pɛlvɪs] *n.* 骨盆

lumbosacral ['lʌmbəu.seikrəl] *adj.* 腰骶的

lumbosacral junction　腰骶连接

erector spinae muscle　竖脊肌

torques ['tɔrkwɪz] *n.* 力矩

torques equalized　力矩平衡的

twisting [twɪstɪŋ] *n.* 扭转；扭曲

---- **Questions** ----

❶ The atlanto-occipital joint is the joint that allows the skull to move on the vertebral bones. When one stands quietly with his head facing straight forward, which one of the following is the major force to maintain the head in its position?

A. The weight of the head.

B. The weight of the whole body.

C. The strength of the back muscles on the head and neck.

D. The gravity to the head.

❷ When you are standing on tiptoes of your feet, which one of the following joint is the very likely fulcrum for the action?

A. The metatarsophalangeal joint.

B. The subtalar joint.

C. The knee joint.

D. The ankle joint.

❸ Your patient is practicing the biceps curl with a 2-kilograms dumbbell. Based on what you learned, which one of the following is the resistance in this case?

A. The strength of the biceps brachii muscle.

B. The 2-kilogram dumbbell.

C. The strength of the triceps brachii muscle.

D. The elbow joint.

❹ In comparison of the size of the base of support (BOS), which one of the following has the largest BOS?

A. Standing on both feet–both are separated in a shoulder distance.

B. Standing on both feet–both feet's medial sides are close to each other.

C. Standing on both feet–one foot is in front of other foot along a straight line.

D. Standing on one foot.

❺ When you are holding a heavy box in front of you, which one of the following is correct about the main resistance, the primary force, and the fulcrum?

A. Resistance–the box, force–back muscles, fulcrum–the lumbosacral joint (L5–S1 joint).

B. Resistance–abdominal muscles, force–back muscles, fulcrum–the lumbosacral joint (L5–S1 joint).

C. Resistance–back muscles, force–abdominal muscles, fulcrum–the lumbosacral joint (L5–S1 joint).

D. Resistance–the box, force–abdominal muscles, fulcrum–the lumbosacral joint (L5–S1 joint).

Answers

❶ C ❷ A ❸ B ❹ A ❺ A

Rehabilitation Professionals
康复专业人员

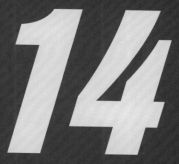

Among rehabilitation professionals, there are often rehabilitation physicians (also known as physiatrists), physical therapists, occupational therapists, speech therapists, and rehabilitation nurses. Physiatrists are medical specialists that usually work in (acute hospitals) inpatient settings or rehabilitation hospitals and provide general medical and rehabilitation-specialty management for patients with a variety of disabilities. Physiatrists maintain patients' medical stability and prevent patients from secondary disability. They do not usually perform surgical operations but they do conduct many procedures for the diagnosis and treatment of spasticity, pain, and medical problems resulting from stroke, spinal cord injury, traumatic brain injury, osteoarthritis, cerebral palsy, and many others. These procedures may include surface and needle electromyography, nerve conduction testing, musculoskeletal ultrasound, joint or trigger point injections, platelet rich plasma injections, acupuncture,

在康复专业人员中，常包括康复医师（也被称为物理治疗医师）、物理治疗师、作业治疗师、言语治疗师和康复护士。康复医师通常是在（综合性医院）住院部或康复专科医院为各种残疾患者提供常规医务和康复专科治疗的专业医师。康复医师要维持患者的病情稳定并防止患者出现继发性残疾。他们一般不进行外科手术，但是会进行关于脑卒中、脊髓损伤、脑外伤、骨关节炎、脑性瘫痪和其他疾病所导致的痉挛、疼痛和其他病症的诊断和治疗方面的操作。这些操作包括表面和针刺肌电图、神经传导测试、肌骨超声、关节内或者扳机点注射、富含血小板血浆注射、针灸、鞘内巴氯芬泵以及抗痉挛药的使用。在一个康复治疗团队中，康复医师通常是协调团队成员工作的领导者。所有成员相互合作，而不是谁为谁服务。

intrathecal baclofen pumps, and use of anti-spasticity drugs. In a rehabilitation team, the physiatrist is often the leader that coordinates the team members' activities. All members work with each other, rather than for each other.

Physical therapists (PTs) are highly educated healthcare professionals who provide rehabilitation services to relieve pain, restore function, and improve mobility without using any surgical procedures or medical prescriptions. Interventions that PTs provide include the use of physical modalities, therapeutic exercises, and the use of hands-on skills. Modalities may include hot/cold packs, electrical stimulation, therapeutic ultrasound, iontophoresis, laser therapy, and aquatic therapy. Therapeutic exercises may include those that are able to reduce pain and improve strength, flexibility, balance, endurance, and gait ability. Hands-on manipulative skills may include the Bobath technique, proprioceptive neuromuscular facilitation (PNF), Mulligan skills, Maitland skills, muscle energy techniques and many others. Subspecialties in physical therapy include neurology, orthopedics, sports, cardiorespiratory, pediatrics, geriatrics, women's health, and oncology. Physical therapists usually work in acute hospitals, rehabilitation hospitals, nursing homes, outpatient rehabilitation clinics, home health agencies, fitness centers, and sports team facilities.

Occupational therapists (OTs) are very important members in the rehabilitation

物理治疗师是受过高等教育的医疗保健人员，通过非外科手术或非药物治疗方式为患者提供缓解疼痛、恢复功能及改善活动性等康复服务。物理治疗师的干预方式包括物理因子治疗、运动疗法和手法治疗。物理因子治疗包括热/冷疗、电疗、超声波治疗、直流电离子导入法、激光疗法和水疗。运动疗法包括可减轻疼痛，提高肌力、灵活性、平衡、耐受性和步行能力的运动锻炼。手法治疗可能包括Bobath（神经发育）技术、本体感觉神经肌肉促通技术（PNF）、Mulligan技术、Maitland技术、肌肉能量技术和许多其他技术。物理治疗学（PT）的亚专业包括神经的、骨科的、运动学的、心肺的、儿科的、老年的、妇女健康的和肿瘤学的。物理治疗师通常在综合性医院、康复医院、护理院、康复门诊、上门服务的居家康护机构、健身中心和运动队工作。

作业治疗师在康复治疗团

profession. They mainly work with patients to restore their abilities to perform activities of daily living (ADLs) and instrumental activities of daily living (IADLs). ADLs are basic functions that a person performs at home without assistance. Examples of ADLs include eating, personal hygiene (such as brushing your teeth, washing your face, combing your hair, etc.), bathing, dressing, toileting, and transferring (such as from the bed to a chair). IADLs are activities that a person can do that makes him or her able to independently live in a community. Examples of IADLs include house cleaning, meal preparation, shopping for needed items, personal financial management, and participation in community activities. OTs will perform a thorough assessment of a patient's physical, mental, emotional, and/or developmental aspects as well as the patient's living or working environment. They will then use this information to integrate components of daily activities into the intervention plan in order to help the patient reach his or her goals for ADLs and IADLs. OTs usually work in the same clinical settings as PTs but very few work in fitness centers and sports team facilities.

Speech-language pathologists (SLPs), often referred to as speech therapists (STs), evaluate and treat patients with dysfunctions in speech, language, communication, and swallowing. More specifically, STs often see patients who have difficulty with correct and fluent speech, show disorders in expressing or understanding language, choose inappropriate

队中是非常重要的成员。他们主要帮助患者重获进行日常生活活动和工具性日常生活活动的能力。日常生活活动能力是一个人在无人帮助的情况下独自在家中生活的基本能力。日常生活活动能力的范例包括吃饭、个人卫生（例如刷牙、洗脸、梳头发等）、洗澡、穿衣、如厕和转移（例如床椅转移）。工具性日常生活活动能力指可以帮助患者在社区中独立生存的能力。工具性日常生活活动能力的范例包括打扫房间、准备食物、购买所需物品、个人财物管理和社区活动参与。作业治疗师们会对患者的肢体、心理、情感和/或生长发育能力进行评估，也会对患者的生活或工作环境进行评估。他们接下来会利用这些信息将日常生活活动整合到治疗计划中去，从而帮助患者达到获得日常生活活动能力和工具性日常生活活动能力的目标。作业治疗师们通常在和物理治疗师一样的临床机构中工作，但很少在健身中心和运动队工作。

语言病理学家，通常被称为言语治疗师，为患者的言语障碍、表达障碍、交流障碍和吞咽障碍进行评估和治疗。更具体地说，言语治疗师面对的一般是在正确或流畅说话方面存在困难，在表达和理解方面出现混乱，选择错误语言文字或非语言

verbal words or non-verbal communication behaviors, or exert deficits in organizing thoughts, paying attention, and keeping memory. Further, swallowing disorders (dysphagia), such as difficulties with feeding and swallowing, are also one of the main areas that STs deal with. Usually, STs work in the same settings as OTs.

Rehabilitation nurses (RNs) are nurses with a subspecialty in rehabilitation skills and in working with patients who are suffering from disability and cannot function well physically and/or mentally. They are able to execute prescriptions from physicians like positioning patients properly, handling bladder dysfunction, dealing with dysphagia, assisting in the treatment of spasticity, and many others. In addition, they may also be able to identify deficits in functional mobility (strength, flexibility, endurance, balance, posture, and gait) as well as in performance of ADLs and IADLs. RNs work with therapists in all kinds of clinical settings to improve patients' functionality for daily life.

Many hands-on care medical professionals are frequently considered to be part of the orthopedic rehabilitation profession. Osteopathic doctors received both medical and osteopathic manipulative treatment (OMT) training in schools in the US, or just OMT training in other western countries. They use their hands to holistically treat pain from the musculoskeletal system as well as from internal organs. Chiropractors use their hands and modalities to manipulate or "adjust" patients who may have alignment problems of

文字交流行为，或在组织思维、集中注意力和保持记忆方面存在缺陷的患者。再者，吞咽障碍（吞咽困难）者，例如存在进食和吞咽障碍的患者也是言语治疗师的主要负责领域之一。通常来讲，言语治疗师和作业治疗师在相同的机构中工作。

康复护士是具备康复护理能力的护士们，他们面对的主要是存在残疾和在肢体或心理方面存在功能障碍的患者。他们可以执行康复医师的治疗处方，例如患者的正确姿势摆放、处理膀胱功能障碍、处理吞咽困难、协助治疗痉挛及许多其他方面的工作。此外，他们也可以识别功能活动性方面（如力量、灵活性、耐力、平衡、姿势和步态）的缺陷，还有一般日常活动能力和工具性日常活动能力的不足。康复护士和治疗师一起在各类临床机构中工作，帮助患者提高日常生活活动能力。

许多时候徒手治疗医师通常被看作是骨科康复专业的重要组成。整骨医师在美国要在学校接受医学专业知识和整骨疗法（OMT）培训，而在其他西方国家或只接受过OMT培训。他们会用双手整体性地治疗肌肉骨骼系统以及内脏器官方面的疼痛。整脊师用他们的手法和治疗仪器来处理或调整患者存在的脊椎或身体力线问题从而减轻痛苦，改善功能。中国的

the spine and/or body parts in order to alleviate pain and improve function. Tui-Na doctors in China can also be in this category. They treat patients with hands-on care based on theories of traditional Chinese medicine (e.g., the acupuncture points and meridians).

推拿医师也属于此类范畴，他们通过基于传统中医理论（如针灸穴位和经络）的治疗手法对患者进行治疗。

New words

rehabilitation professionals 康复专业人员

physician [fɪ'zɪʃən] *n.* 医师

physiatrist [ˌfɪzɪ'ætrɪst] *n.* 康复医师

physical therapist 物理治疗师

occupational Therapist 作业治疗师

speech therapist 言语治疗师

specialist ['spɛʃəlɪst] *n.* 专家；专科医师

inpatient ['ɪnpeʃənt] *n.* 住院患者

spasticity [spæs'tɪsətɪ] *n.* 痉挛

traumatic [traʊ'mætɪk] *adj.*（生理）外伤的；创伤的

traumatic brain injury 创伤性脑损伤

osteoarthritis ['ɑstɪoɑr'θraɪtɪs] *n.* 骨关节炎

electromyography [ɪˌlɛktromaɪ'ɑgrəfɪ] *n.* 肌电描记术；肌电图

musculoskeletal ultrasound 肌肉骨骼超声

platelet rich plasma injections 富血小板血浆注射

acupuncture ['ækjupʌŋktʃɚ] *n.* 针刺；针刺疗法

intrathecal [ˌɪntrə'θiːkəl] *adj.* 鞘内，髓鞘内

baclofen [bæk'ləufən] *n.* 巴氯芬

intrathecal baclofen pumps 鞘内巴氯芬泵

oral anti-spasticity 口服抗痉挛药

restore [rɪ'stɔr] *vt.* 恢复；修复 *vi.* 恢复；还原

prescription [prɪ'skrɪpʃən] *n.* 药方

intervention *n.* 干预，干涉；处置

modality [mo'dæLətɪ] *n.* 物理因子（疗法）

iontophoresis [aɪˌɔntəufə'riːsɪs] *n.* 电离子透入疗法；离子电渗疗法

aquatic [ə'kwætɪk] *adj.* 水生的；在水中或水面进行的

endurance [ɪn'dʊrəns] *n.* 耐力

manipulative [mə'nɪpjələtɪv] *adj.* 巧妙处理的；操纵的，用手控制的

Bobath technique　　Bobath 技术

proprioceptive [ˌprəʊprɪəu'septɪv] *adj.* 本体感受的

facilitation [fəˌsɪlə'teʃən] 易化技术；促通技术

proprioceptive neural facilitation　　本体感受的神经促通技术

Mulligan skills　　Mulligan 技术

Maitland skills　　Maitland 技术

subspecialty ['sʌb.speʃəltɪ] *n.* 亚专业

orthopedics [ˌɔrθə'pɪdɪks] *n.* 矫形（外科），骨科

cardiorespiratory [ˌkɑrdɪorɪs'paɪrətərɪ] *adj.* 心肺的

pediatrics [ˌpɪdɪ'ætrɪks] *n.* 小儿科

geriatrics [ˌdʒɛrɪ'ætrɪks] *n.* 老年病学；老年病科

oncology [ɑn'kɑlədʒɪ] *n.* 肿瘤科，肿瘤学

outpatient ['aʊt'peʃənt] *n.* 门诊患者

outpatient rehabilitation clinics　　门诊康复诊所

home health agencies　　居家康护机构

fitness center　　健身中心；健身房

sports team facilities　　运动队训练处（场馆）

instrumental [ˌɪnstrə'mɛntl] *adj.* 乐器的；有帮助的；器具的

 instrumental activities of daily living　　工（器）具性日常生活活动

personal hygiene　　个人卫生

integrate ['ɪntɪgret] *vt.* 使……完整；使……成整体

pathologist [pə'θɑlədʒɪst] *n.* 病理学家

speech-language pathologist　　言语障碍治疗师

execute ['ɛksɪkjut] *vt.* 实行；执行；处死

dysphagia [dɪs'fedʒɪə] *n.* 吞咽困难

holistically　　整体地；全面地

chiropractor ['kaɪərопræktə] 整脊治疗师

alignment [ə'laɪnmənt] *n.* 成直线；校准

acupuncture points and meridians　　穴位和经络

---------------------------- Questions ----------------------------

1 In clinical rehabilitation settings, physiatrists are often referred to _____.
  A. physical therapists   B. occupational therapists
  C. psychiatrists   D. rehabilitation physicians

2 Among the rehabilitation interventions, which one of them is the intervention that a physical therapist or physiotherapist does not provide?
  A. Therapeutic exercises.   B. Physical modalities.
  C. Platelet rich plasma injections.   D. Hands-on manipulation.

3 Which one of the following activities is considered as a content of the instrumental activities of daily living (IADL), rather than a content of the ADL?
  A. Brushing teeth.   B. Using toilet.
  C. Cooking a meal.   D. Transferring from bed to a chair.

4 Which one of the following rehabilitation professions has the more expertise than others for treating patients with dysphagia?
  A. The rehabilitation nurse.   B. The physical therapist.
  C. The occupational therapist.   D. The speech therapist.

5 In a rehabilitation hospital or department, a patient with spinal cord injury is suffered from bladder dysfunction. On a daily basis, such a dysfunction is usually watched and taken care by a _____.
  A. rehabilitation nurse   B. physical therapist
  C. occupational therapist   D. speech therapist

Answers

1 A   **2** C   **3** C   **4** D   **5** A

Description of A Geriatric Case for Rehabilitation

老年康复病例的描述

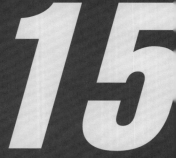

15

A 79-year-old female was referred to rehabilitation therapy for evaluation and treatment due to two falls in the last 7 days at home. The falls did not cause severe traumatic injury to her, but caught the attention of her children. Prior to admission, the patient was able to ambulate on a level surface with a cane (walking stick) about 75 to 100 meters independently. She began to feel more fatigued and demonstrated unsteady gait about two weeks before her first fall.

This patient currently lived alone in a senior living center. She is the mother of 3 children and the grandmother of 4 grandchildren. She had a past medical history of hypertension, congestive heart failure, and anxiety for over five years, and also occasional urinary incontinence for about 3 weeks. Besides the above, no other past neurological, vascular, endocrinological, psychological, or infectious problems were raised.

One of her daughters stated that her mom did not exercise much, liked watching TV, and

一名79岁的女性因在家中最近7天内两次跌倒而被转介到康复治疗部进行评估和治疗。虽然跌倒并没有造成患者严重的创伤，但是却引起了患者孩子们的重视。在入院前患者还是能够独立地用手杖在水平的路面上行走75～100米。她大约在第一次跌倒的前2周开始感到更加疲惫并且出现步态不稳。

该患者目前独居于一个老年居住中心。她有3个孩子和4个孙辈。她有超过5年的高血压、充血性心力衰竭和焦虑症的既往史，且近3周来偶有尿失禁。除此之外，既往无其他神经、血管、内分泌、心理或传染性疾病史。

其女之一述：患者不喜运

could sit on her couch for hours. There were no family and genetic diseases among their family members and siblings. This patient was a pleasant, but sometimes confused, lady. She had no history of alcohol and tobacco use and also had no known drug allergies. A recent chest X-ray revealed cardiomegaly, no pulmonary infiltrate, and no pleural effusion. Her current list of medications was available and checked.

Physical Examination. Vital signs: temperature: 37.3 deg Celsius, pulse rate: 68 beat/min, respiratory rate: 16 breaths/min; blood pressure: 130/77 mmHg. The patient was moderately obese, lethargic, and confused on occasion with time and place. She sat in a chair with a slouching posture. No dyspnea at rest was noticed. Extremities were without cyanosis and clubbing. Sensory and tendon reflexes were intact bilaterally. Manual muscle strength testing revealed 2/5 for bilateral upper extremities and 3/5 for biateral lower extremities. She needed no assistance for bed mobility; contact guard for therapeutic activities, transfering, and static sitting; and minimal assistance for ambulation for 10 meters with a rolling walker. The patient's goal was to return to her apartment and walk 75–100 meters independently on a level surface again when discharged.

Brief Description of Intervention and Discharge Plans. After the physical examination, the generalized weakness was thought to be a combined result of complications from a sedentary lifestyle and medical conditions. These

动,喜欢看电视,在沙发上一坐就是几个小时。他们的家庭成员和兄弟姐妹中没有家族和遗传疾病史。患者是一位愉悦但有时有些糊涂的女士。她没有烟酒史,也没有已知的药物过敏。最近的一次胸部X线检查显示心脏扩大,没有肺部浸润,也没有胸腔积液。她目前的药物清单是可供查阅的。

体格检查。生命体征:体温37.30℃,脉率68次/分,呼吸频率16次/分,血压130/77 mmHg。患者中度肥胖,昏昏欲睡,偶尔对时间和地点会糊涂。她以懒散的姿势坐在椅子上。休息时无呼吸困难。四肢无发绀和杵状指。双侧感觉和腱反射无异常。手动肌肉测试结果显示双侧上肢为2/5,双侧下肢为3/5。她床上活动不需要帮助;治疗活动、转移和静坐时需要有人扶着(contact guard);使用滚轮助行器行走10米的距离时需要少量的帮助(minimal assistance)。患者的目标是在出院后她能返回她的老年公寓,并再次能在水平路面上独立行走75～100米。

康复干预和出院计划简介。体检后,患者的全身虚弱被认为是基于久坐不动的生活方式加上其疾病情况共同导致的并发性的综合结果。康复治疗干

therapeutic interventions would be co-conducted by both physical and occupational therapists in a functionally oriented format, including daily strengthening, endurance, balance, and gait training in combination with cognitive training in the therapy hall: 45 minutes each session for 4 weeks. The therapy would be within the parallel bars during the first week, using a rolling walker to walk about 50 meters during the second week, 50 meters with a small quad cane for third week, and 75 meters with the small quad cane independently and be able to perform some dual-tasks while walking during the fourth week. Also, a home visit to identify potential risks of falls at home and a patient education session with family members (including discussion of an individualized home exercise program) should be done by the end of the fourth week.

预将由物理治疗师和作业治疗师以功能导向的形式在治疗大厅里来共同进行，包括日常的力量、耐力、平衡和步态训练，以及相结合的认知训练：每次45分钟，为期4周。在第1周内，治疗将在双杠内进行，在第2周使用滚轮助行器行走约50米，在第3周使用小四脚拐杖行走50米，在第4周使用小4脚手杖独立行走75米，并能够执行行走时的一些双相任务。此外，应在第4周结束前进行家访，以确定患者在家中跌倒的潜在风险，并与家庭成员进行患者教育（包括讨论个性化的家庭锻炼计划）。

New words

traumatic [traʊˈmætɪk] *adj.* 外伤的，创伤的

admission [ədˈmɪʃən] *n.* 承认；入院

cane [ken] *n.* 手杖

stick [stɪk] *n.* 棍；手杖

fatigued [fəˈtɪgd] *adj.* 疲乏的

demonstrate [ˈdɛmənˈstret] *vt.* 证明，显示

hypertension [ˌhaɪpəˈtɛnʃən] *n.* 高血压

congestive [kənˈdʒɛstɪv] *adj.* 充血的，充血性的

congestive heart failure   充血性心力衰竭

urinary [ˈjʊrənɛrɪ] *adj.* 尿的；泌尿的

incontinence [ɪnˈkɑntɪnəns] *n.* 失禁

vascular [ˈvæskjələ] *adj.* 血管的

endocrinological   内分泌学的

infectious [ɪn'fɛkʃəs] *adj.* 传染的

siblings ['sɪblɪŋz] *n.* 兄弟姐妹；同科

tobacco [tə'bæko] *n.* 烟草

allergy ['ælədʒɪ] *n.* 过敏症

cardiomegaly [ˌkɑrdio'mɛgəlɪ] *n.* 心脏肥大

pulmonary ['pʌlmənɛrɪ] *adj.* 肺的

infiltrate [ɪn'fɪltret] *n.* 渗透物，渗出物

pleural ['pluərə] *adj.* 胸膜的

effusion [ɪ'fjuʒn] *n.* 渗出

pleural effusion　胸膜腔积液

Vital ['vaɪtl] *adj.* 至关重要的；Vital signs 生命体征

Celsius ['sɛlsɪəs] *n.* 摄氏度

respiratory ['rɛspərəˌtɔri] *adj.* 呼吸的

lethargic [lɪ'θɑːdʒɪk] *adj.* 昏睡的；无生气的

slouching ['slautʃɪŋ] *adj.* 懒散的；没精打采的

dyspnea [dɪsp'niə] *n.* 呼吸困难

cyanosis [ˌsaɪə'nosɪs] *n.* 发绀，青紫

clubbing ['klʌbɪŋ] 杵状指

intact [ɪn'tækt] *adj.* 未受损的，正常的

bilaterally [bai'lætərəli] *adv.* 双边地；双方面地

static ['stætɪk] *adj.* 静态的

ambulation [ˌæmbju-'leɪʃən] *n.* 移动；步行

rolling walker　滚轮助行器

discharge [dɪs'tʃɑrdʒ] *n.* v. 批准离开；出院

complication [ˌkɑmplɪ'keʃən] *n.* 并发症

sedentary ['sɛdntɛrɪ] *adj.* 久坐的

oriented ['orɪɛntɪd] *adj.* 导向的

format ['fɔrmæt] *n.* 格式；版式

session ['sɛʃən] *n.* 治疗次数

parallel ['pærəlɛl] *n.* 平行线；*adj.* 平行的；parallel bars　平行双杠

quad cane　四支点拐杖

dual-task　双重任务

---------------------- ❮ **Questions** ❯ ----------------------

❶ What is the primary reason that this patient is referred to rehabilitation therapy?

A. Congestive heart failure.　　　　B. Hypertension.

C. Two falls in the last 7 days.　　　D. Urinary incontinence.

❷ Before being referred to therapy, this patient was able to walk for about 75–100 meters on a level surface with ＿＿＿＿＿.

A. a cane　　　　　　　　　　　B. a pair of crutches

C. a rolling walker　　　　　　　D. a wheelchair

❸ Which one of the following was not identified during the physical examination?

A. Lethargic.　　　　　　　　　B. Confusion.

C. Dyspnea.　　　　　　　　　　D. Obese.

❹ Which one of the following activities does this patient need more assistance than others?

A. Bed mobility.　　　　　　　　B. Transfer.

C. Siting.　　　　　　　　　　　D. Walking.

❺ During 1st week of the therapeutic intervention, the gait training is mainly conducted ＿＿＿＿＿.

A. by using a rolling walker　　　　B. by using a walking stick

C. by using the parallel bars　　　　D. by using the suspension track

Answers ┄┄┄┄┄┄┄┄┄┄┄┄┄┄┄┄┄┄┄┄┄┄┄┄┄┄┄┄┄┄┄┄┄┄┄┄

❶ C　　**❷** A　　**❸** C　　**❹** D　　**❺** C

Patient Interview—Back Pain
患者初诊——背痛

16

Therapist: Hi, Ms. K.

Patient: Hi.

Therapist: My name is Jennifer, your therapist. It's nice to meet you.

Patient: Nice to meet you too.

Therapist: Would you mind if I asked you some questions and did a brief physical exam?

Patient: No, not at all.

Therapist: Great. So what brings you in today?

Patient: I've been having pretty bad back pain.

Therapist: Well, I am glad you came in, so we can take a look and see what's going on. How long has this been a problem?

Patient: Probably about two days.

Therapist: Okay, did anything happen a couple of days ago out of the ordinary?

Patient: I was in a minor car accident.

Therapist: Must have been scary.

Patient: Yeah.

Therapist: What happened?

Patient: I was at a stoplight and the person

治疗师：你好，K女士。

患者：你好。

治疗师：我叫珍妮弗，是你的治疗师，很高兴见到你。

患者：很高兴见到你。

治疗师：你介意我问你一些问题，并做个简短体格检查吗？

患者：不介意。

治疗师：很好，那么，今天你为何而来？

患者：我后背痛得很厉害。

治疗师：哦，我很高兴你能来，这样我们就可以检查一下，确定出了什么问题，后背疼痛持续了多久？

患者：大概两天左右。

治疗师：好的，几天前发生了什么意外的事情吗？

患者：嗯，发生了一起轻微的车祸。

治疗师：一定很吓人。

患者：是的。

治疗师：发生了什么？

患者：嗯，我在等红灯，被身后的

behind me rear-ended me. We weren't going very fast though. I think he was going maybe 5 or 10 miles per hour.

Therapist: Were you wearing your seat belt at the time?

Patient: Yeah.

Therapist: You said you didn't go to the hospital or do any treatment because you didn't feel any pain initially.

Patient: No.

Therapist: When exactly did the pain start? About how many hours after the accident?

Patient: I would probably say 4–6 hours after. I think maybe I was just in shock at first and I didn't really feel any pain or anything.

Therapist: Alright. Where is it bothering you specifically? Can you pinpoint a specific area on your back?

Patient: It is mostly just my back.

Therapist: Both sides?

Patient: Yes.

Therapist: Did you hear any pops or have any numbness or tingling that occurred during the accident?

Patient: No.

Therapist: Is there anything that makes the pain worse?

Patient: Mostly when I bend forward and try to turn my body to the left. It really hurts and feels tight.

Therapist: I noticed that it is very uncomfortable. Is there anything you've noticed that is helping you?

Patient: It helps a little if I take some Ibuprofen and put ice on my back, but it still hurts.

人追尾了。不过速度不快,我想他的速度只有每小时5到10英里。

治疗师: 你当时系安全带了吗?

患者: 系了。

治疗师: 好的,你说因为最初没有感觉到任何疼痛,所以你没有去医院,也没做任何处理?

患者: 是的,没去。

治疗师: 疼痛确切来说是什么时候开始的? 事故发生后大约几个小时?

患者: 我想大概4到6个小时后。我想我刚开始可能只是处于惊吓之中,我没有感觉到任何疼痛或其他不适感。

治疗师: 好的。你具体是后背的哪里痛? 你能指出你后背疼痛的区域吗?

患者: 主要就是后背。

治疗师: 两侧?

患者: 是的。

治疗师: 发生事故时,你有没有听到任何砰砰声,或出现任何麻木或刺痛感?

患者: 没有。

治疗师: 有没有什么情况使疼痛加剧?

患者: 大多数情况下,当我向前弯腰,并向左转腰时,有点疼和紧绷感。

治疗师: 我注意到你的不舒适了,你注意到什么情况下能改善你的症状吗?

患者: 嗯,我吃了一些布洛芬,在后背部放了冰块,这有点帮助,

Therapist: Ok. Can you describe the pain to me?

Patient: It feels like a tight kind of dull pain.

Therapist: Is this pain radiating or moving anywhere?

Patient: Not really. It just goes up and down my back.

Therapist: No pain shooting down to your legs?

Patient: No.

Therapist: On a scale of 1 to 10 with 10 being the worst pain you ever experienced, where would you say you're at now?

Patient: Probably around a 6 or 7 out of 10. Especially when I try to bend forward and turn my head.

Therapist: Is it a constant pain?

Patient: Yes.

Therapist: Since the accident, has your pain been constant or is it getting worse, better?

Patient: It feels it is getting worse, but I don't know if that's just because the Ibuprofen is not working.

Therapist: As far as your past medical history, have you ever had a back or neck injury before?

Patient: No.

Therapist: Ok, let me assist you to get on the exam mat.

Patient: Thank you.

Therapist: Would you please lie face down, on your stomach?

Patient: Sure. I feel tight when I'm turning.

Therapist: Tight when turning left or right?

Patient: Left.

Therapist: Ok. I am pressing on this spot, do

但还是很疼。

治疗师: 好的,你能描述一下你的疼痛吗?

患者: 这感觉像是一种紧绷的隐隐作痛。

治疗师: 这种疼痛是放射的还是移动的?

患者: 不确定,它是在我的后背上下跑动的痛。

治疗师: 腿上没有什么症状吗?

患者: 没有。

治疗师: 从1到10的数值范围里,10是你经历过的最痛的值,你感觉你现在是几分?

患者: 嗯,大概是六七分吧,尤其是当我试图向前弯腰转头的时候。

治疗师: 是持续疼痛吗?

患者: 是的。

治疗师: 事故发生后疼痛是持续的,还是越来越疼,或是越来越好?

患者: 感觉越来越糟,但我不知道是不是只是因为布洛芬已经不起作用了。

治疗师: 就你过去的病史而言,你以前有过背部或颈部受伤的经历吗?

患者: 没有。

治疗师: 好的,让我来帮你上检查垫吧。

患者: 谢谢。

治疗师: 请你脸朝下趴着好吗?

患者: 当然可以,我转身时觉得很紧。

治疗师: 向左转还是向右转时觉得紧?

患者: 向左转时。

治疗师: 好的,我按压这个部位,

you feel more pain?

Patient: No, still the same.

Therapist: Now would you please raise this leg like so and hold it right here, don't let me push it down.

Patient: Wow, haha that's difficult.

Therapist: Ok, now I'm going to push your leg in different directions and I want you to hold it when I do so.

Patient: Ok, go ahead.

Therapist: Thank you.

你觉得疼吗？

患者：不，一样。

治疗师：现在请你把这条腿像这样抬起来，停在这儿控制住，别让我把它往下推动了。

患者：哇，哈哈，这很难。

治疗师：好的，现在我要把你的腿往不同的方向推，我要你在我这样做的时候控住你的腿。

患者：好的，开始做吧。

治疗师：谢谢。

New words

numbness [nʌmnəs] *n.* 麻木

tingle ['tɪŋgl] *n.* 刺痛

ibuprofen [ˌaɪbjuˈprofɛn] *n.* 布洛芬（抗炎，镇痛药）